AN
80
YEAR
OLD
DOCTOR'S
SECRETS
OF
POSITIVE
HEALTH

AN
80
YEAR
OLD
DOCTOR'S
SECRETS
OF
POSITIVE
HEALTH

by

William Brady, M.D.

PRENTICE-HALL, INC.

Englewood Cliffs, N.J.

First printing. . . . .*July, 1961*
Second printing. . . . .*October, 1961*

Library of Congress Catalog Card Number:
61-1200

Printed in the United States of America
24689—T

PREFACE: SINGULAR NOTIONS OF A HORSE—AND—BUGGY DOCTOR

If you are afraid you're going mad you are probably quite sane. On the other hand, if you have really lost some of your marbles, you will be the last to know it. I have found this to be true throughout my professional lifetime. As a passing observation it used to amuse me, but now that I'm a doddering octogenarian I confess it begins to worry me.

Especially so since the *Journal of the American Medical Association* once had this to say about me editorially:

"Among the newspaper columnists who inform the public on matters of health is Dr. William Brady, formerly of Elmira, N.Y. and now of Buffalo in the same state. Dr. Brady has published columns which have seemed to many physicians exceptionally sound as to the advice rendered and the facts stated. He has occasionally departed into strange notions which seemed excusable on the ground that they seemed designed to attract popular attention without doing serious harm. For example, he has promoted strongly the notion that daily somersaults in bed are an excellent technic for keeping the body in health . . ."

I was thinking about this—and about how easy it is to be misquoted—while doing my own daily rolls this morning. I wondered if as a result of reading the *Journal* piece anybody did try to turn somersaults in bed, and whether the poor gink who attempted it blamed me for the consequences. For myself, though I have been rolling 'em for forty years, I always do it on the ground or the floor. Never had the courage to try a bed!

Until now I have always stressed the physiological benefits one derives from daily somersaulting, but this morning it occurred to me that at eighty you get an extra benefit of incalculable value— the psychological satisfaction of knowing you are not decrepit. I suppose this doesn't mean much to callow sexagenarians, but just wait a few more years and you'll see.

The medical profession generally regards any departure from its accepted ways as "strange notions." Many of my teachings have been so branded by my quondam fellows in the AMA. I don't mind, so long as they don't gang up on me along with the devital- ized-food and the prescription-nostrum merchants to silence me altogether. For my "strange notions," based as they are on a life- time of sometimes unorthodox observation and practice, *are geared to keeping patients out of doctors' offices*. I have always been con- cerned with health rather than illness and this book is a further attempt in the same direction.

William Brady, M.D.

Contents

AN
80
YEAR
OLD
DOCTOR'S
SECRETS
OF
POSITIVE
HEALTH

Chapter One

SEVEN KEYS TO VITE

THE SECRET OF LIFE-LONG YOUTHFULNESS

Moses was 120 years old when he died; Noah was 950; Jared lived to be 962 and all the days of Methuselah were 969 years.

There is good reason to believe that the Biblical patriarchs reckoned their ages differently—possibly by seasons. After all, man's life span could not have changed so radically over a mere few thousand years. In fact the late brilliant, but eccentric, Woods Hutchinson, once wrote a series of articles in which he strongly implied that people claiming to be over a hundred had lost count of their years or were too fond of publicity. I am neutral in the controversy, and besides, I feel everyone is entitled to lie a little about his or her age. But the fact remains that every once in a while we do come across a man or woman who is very, very old, and then invariably people want to know what their recipe is for long life.

It doesn't really matter what your calendar age happens to be. It might in fact be better all around to forget one's chronological age and consider only the anatomical or physiological age. Longevity is really a vascular question—"A man is as old as his arteries." As Sir William Osler, the great Canadian medical teacher and writer, pointed out long ago, "A man of twenty-eight or -nine may have the arteries of a man of sixty, a man of forty may present vessels as much degenerated as they should be at eighty . . ."

Osler used the word *degenerated*. He did not say precisely what he meant, but Webster and standard medical dictionaries define degeneration clearly enough:

1. "Deterioration: a change from a higher to a lower form; especially change of tissue to a lower or less functionally active form. When there is chemical change of the tissue itself, it is true degeneration; when the change consists in the deposit of abnormal matter in the tissues, it is infiltration."   (Dorland)
2. "A retrogressive pathological change in cells or tissues in consequence of which the functioning power is lost and the living substance becomes converted into an inert mass." (Stedman)
3. "Deterioration of a tissue or an organ in which its vitality is diminished; substitution of a lower for a higher form of structure, either by chemical change of the tissue (true degeneration) or the deposit of abnormal matter in the tissue (infiltration)."   (Webster)

Dorland and Webster, with their jargon about "deposit of abnormal matter in the tissues," carefully adhere to what the old-time doctors "done tole 'em." In my opinion this is childish credulity and the definition calls for drastic revision.

Stedman's definition of degeneration as a medical term needs only one minor revision: instead of saying "functioning power is lost" it would be more accurate to say it is *impaired*. For once it is truly lost—well, may the poor soul rest in peace.

The medical pundits of the nineteenth century had a habit of making pronouncements about things being thus and so—and none ventured to question or reject their verdicts. Indeed there was no way of gathering scientific evidence to refute them. Today this has changed. All theories of "deposit of abnormal matter in the tissues" to the contrary, it has never been satisfactorily demonstrated that foreign or abnormal matter is ever deposited in the tissues. This applies to all such excess matter as fat, calcium, cholesterol or whatever: their presence in the tissues is a *consequence* of degeneration, a patchwork that's the best nature can do after the capacity to produce functionally active cells has failed. The old notion of "infiltration," the dumping of "abnormal matter" in worn out,

aging or dying tissue or organ is, as we are finding out, for the birds
—the dodo birds.

The reason the modern merchants of medicine, as I call them,
continue to peddle this idea to their customers, is that there is tremendous profit in it. The doctor who keeps his patient on a low-
cholesterol diet does him no harm, of course. But I venture to
remind him that even if the cholesterol in the blood is brought
below an arbitrary "normal" level and kept there, this still has no
effect on the condition of the heart or arteries. So where do we go
from here? Clearly, the problem is to *prevent* deterioration before it
sets in rather than try to cope with it later on.

A shadowy figure of the 15th century named Luigi Cornaro
lived to be 102 and wrote a book, *The Art of Living Long,* coun-
selling what we consider sound principles—moderation in eating
and temperance in everything. Then there was George Cheyne, a
Scot born in 1671, who by the age of thirty had attained the moun-
tainous weight of 448 pounds, set about reducing, shed nearly 300
pounds of blubber by dieting, lived in fine fettle well into his seventies and wrote an essay on diet which has become something of a
classic. One of his axioms, quoted by Dr. Osler in his *Practice,*
reads:

> Every wise man, after Fifty, ought to begin to lessen at least
> the quaintity of his aliment (food) and if he would continue free
> of great and dangerous Distempers and preserve his Sense and
> Faculties clear to the last he ought every seven years [seven is
> the magic number, remember] go on abating gradually and
> sensibly, and at last descend out of Life as he ascended into it,
> even unto a Child's Diet.

"Milk and Sweet Sound Blood," he says elsewhere, "differ in
nothing but in Color: Milk is Blood."

Whether or not one agrees with everything that good old George
had to say, he, like Cornaro, comes to the conclusion that moderation in eating and temperance in everything are the key to long
life and health. Come to think about it, all the nonegenarians and
nearly all the octogenarians I know are abstemious. Chances are,
too, that whether by design or by instinct their routine includes a
balanced diet. But, of that, more presently.

The secret of long life is closely connected with something for which, with the collaboration of readers of my syndicated health column years ago, I coined a new word—V I T E. Vite rhymes with kite. Lest you confuse it with the French *vite,* which means "quickly," just remember that the French word is an adverb and it rhymes with Pete.

Here is my definition of V I T E :

> Vite means preservation of the characteristics of youth, better-than-average nutritional condition as manifested in lower death-rates, better growth and development, extension of the prime of life in both directions, material improvement of the life expectation of adults, higher average level of positive health throughout the life cycle, greater pep, more vitality, the highest degree of natural immunity, an adequate fund of reserve power to tide over emergencies and strains, the resiliency of the untamed animal or the primitive savage.

You see, it implies much more than just "not complaining." Yes, if you like, it means being lively, sprightly, animated, spirited, with vigor, vivacity, zeal. A man or animal with vite is nimble, capable, eager to play, ready to fight or run away. Please don't assume that the definition of vite is a mere collection of idle phrases. Every idea touched on is based on much study of the subject. Nothing idle about it. I tell you vite is a priceless thing, and yet almost everybody, if he wishes, can add a little bit more to what he already has and the gain is bound to be manifest in one respect or another, as suggested by the definition.

Vite is the difference between the individual who is "not complaining" and the one who enjoys being alive.

Vite is a "higher average level of positive health." Now please don't think of Prof. Musclebound strutting around in his leopard-skin costume and telling the customers how puny he was ten years ago and how his six easy lessons by mail will give anybody a superb collection of bumps like this. That sort of thing has nothing to do with vite. Rather the overdevelopment of muscles tends to lower vite.

The positive health associated with vite is a state of perfect or nearly perfect functional efficiency which few "well" people enjoy, mainly because they are ignorant of the seven keys to vite which will be presented here in due course.

As a rule, the rating of the indivdual who considers himself or herself well or in good health is actually around 75 or 80 per cent. It is usually not difficult for such an individual, if he or she knows the seven keys and uses them, to boost his or her standing to 90 per cent or more.

Altogether there are four main levels of health. On the lowest level, of course, are people who are ill of one or another chronic disease. Next higher are people who feel "poorly" or complain a good deal but perhaps have no definite disease or drift along aimlessly because they do not think a proper medical examination and diagnosis necessary. On the third level are the great majority of the seventy-five percenters content to make the grade who think, if they ever give the matter any consideration, that such health as they do have is a matter of chance or fortune and one may as well leave well enough alone. Finally, up on the top level, are the 90 percenters who have found some of the keys to vite and used them.

In the era of pathological anatomy, in the Gay Nineties, doctors concerned themselves chiefly with "organic" disease, morbid changes they could detect by physical examination. They gave scant consideration to subjective evidence, the complaints or symptoms that brought patients to the doctor. And so gran'pa or grandma had some justification for hesitating to bother the doctor with their minor ailments. And perhaps the old-time practitioner sincerely believed he was giving what we now call good psychotherapy, wholesome reassurance, when he listened with the stethoscope, percussed the chest, palpated a few likely spots and dismissed the patient with a laugh and a remark that he only wished he might enjoy health as good.

What did a formal physical examination cost in those days? From $2 to $5. It included whatever the doctor could learn by sight (inspection), touch (palpation) and hearing (percussion and auscultation). A periodic health examination today costs $25 plus —plus fees for whatever specific laboratory, chemical or microscopic tests that the individual's occupation or environment may indicate, or tests that the individual's symptoms may suggest.

Readers often ask just what a periodic physical or medical examination or health test should include and I have no precise answer, but in any case I can say this: If I were the examinee I wouldn't pay for any fashionable business such as determination of cholesterol level in blood, measurement of uric acid in blood, estimation of metabolism rate with a Rube Goldberg gadget (metabolimeter, used in basal metabolism test) and other superfluities. These frills may impress the gullible with the belief that his medic is as scientific as all getout, but in my opinion they have little value.

On the other hand, today anyone who harbors the notion that one must have something definite to complain about before seeing a doctor—else the doctor will laugh at you—ought to have his head examined, not only his body. There is no need to drift aimlessly in a borderland of *malaise* when there are competent physicians available for proper examination and diagnosis. This is not only a question of providing for early detection of serious illness. In 95 cases out of a 100 the problem is simply to raise your own standard of health in a world where from childhood our over-civilized way of life has been stacking the cards against you, partly because of the diet it imposes on you and your fellow-Americans and partly because of your work and play habits and the very air you breathe.

After World War I there was considerable agitation in favor of health and physical education in the public schools. In some communities attendance of gymnasium classes became compulsory and here and there graduation from high school required proficiency in swimming.

But this turn toward liberal education never was accepted by the old-timers. They looked down their noses upon physical education from the very first. They treated the health and physical instructors as triflers with the serious business of training youth. Thanks to the laziness of all growing children and the ignorance and indifference of most parents, health and physical education in most public schools became a farce indeed. Some principals curry favor with some parents and the local sporting fraternity by calling assemblies of the pupils to extract substantial contributions for the purchase of equipment for the team and to impress upon them the importance of attending the big game and screaming hysterically at the direction of the leader. This make-believe is about all the physical education the majority of schoolboys and schoolgirls are getting today.

When I compare the condition of growing children today, especially the children in towns and cities, with that of growing children when I was one on Chapel Street in Canandaigua in the Finger Lakes region of Western New York—I feel sorry for them. If they try to play in the street somebody calls the police. As for formal playgrounds, if the community provides any they are usually so far from home that a kid gets to use 'em only occasionally. Even getting to school and getting home isn't much fun any more. *Riding* in automobiles, busses, streetcars, and subways, is depriving youngsters of the benefits and the fun they should get walking to and from school and in horse-chestnut, snowball or fistic encounters with kids from other schools along the way.

There were two such schools along the way when I was a boy in Canandaigua. First, the parochial school on Main Street, where the Catholic church now stands. The parochial school boys were about our own age and always eager for a fight. Then there was the old Academy farther North on Main Street, a private boarding school for boys. Some of them seemed, we thought, to consider themselves a cut above ordinary public school or parochial school boys—and so we Catholics and Protestants sometimes declared temporary truce among ourselves to gang up on the snooty lads when we outnumbered them.

There was absolutely no physical education in our public school. Nevertheless I believe boys, at least, derived more benefit from *play* out of school than boys today get from what purports to be physical education in school.

How many growing boys today ever learn how it feels to get "second wind?"

How many American schoolboys can chin themselves? Studies by health and education authorities recently showed that most European schoolboys can chin themselves and most American schoolboys can't.

We Chapel Street kids used to get "second wind" somewhere

between the Episcopal Church and the Red Jacket Club, when we
were running to fires, which usually occurred somewhere down
below the tracks. It was a wonderful feeling! Most of us could chin
ourselves, stand and walk on our hands, turn somersaults (we
called 'em airsprings) and jump over any hedge along Main Street.
The whole neighborhood was our playground, and rarely did anybody venture to complain to the police.

Today this privilege has gone with the dirt roads. A lot of boys
in their early 'teens are pretty boys and carry pocket combs to
prove it. They can no more do a forward roll and come up on their
feet smiling than can their fathers. I feel sorry for these kids. All
they need is a fair break, which they are not likely to get in towns
and cities where there is no room for playgrounds, parks, baseball
diamonds, athletic fields, sand lots, where any acreage that might
provide recreation is generally snapped up by the real estate interests before the municipality can take a reluctant step to acquire it.
Today if a boy wants to play he has to arrange in advance and
make a project out of it—and so have the joy taken out of the
game. No wonder he loses interest and spends his spare time in the
sweet shop, the movies, watching TV, or reading the funnies.

This is no kind of start to be given in life and if that's how *you*
grew up you doubtless need a boost to begin living at whatever
happens to be the optimum level for you. This is where V I T E
can help you. I offer you, with my best wishes, to use in your everyday life seven keys which I shall discuss in chapters to follow.
They are, not necessarily in the order of their importance:

> Temperance
> Rejuvenation Diet
> Correct Breathing
> Iodine Ration
> Vitamin Feeding
> Exercise
> Nudity (not to be confused with nudism!)
> Conservation of the Teeth

Chapter Two

GOOD TEETH FOR GOOD HEALTH

Just as I was starting to attend school at the age of five, under the sainted Miss Lutie Berner, my father retired from black-smithing because of an injury and was serving as janitor at Chapel Street School at a wage of $8.00 a month. He kept the job a long time. As though it were last summer I remember him in his hexagonal flag shanty at the railroad crossing on W. Gibson Street (a landmark long since gone) trying to make me understand that *all disease begins with the stomach.*

When I was a sophomore medical student I disagreed, but now I think my father was not so far wrong. Briefly, my reasoning is this: Most of the common and garden varieties of complaints for which people keep "trying" this or that medicine, diet, drugless therapy and what not, are manifestations of nutritional deficiency. But I am prone to carry my father's dictum further. *Most disease begins in the mouth,* with impairment of nutrition due to faulty digestion. *Neglect of the teeth* and *loss of teeth* are universal factors of nutritional deficiency, or malnutrition, in this country of ours.

You can see why I consider sound teeth, whether your own or store-bought, one of the essentials if you are going to have V I T E.

Mastication of food is essential for good digestion, and proper mastication requires a full complement of functionally efficient teeth. Yankeeland being in some ways still a free country, you are entitled to show your ignorance if you wish by dismissing this as one of my peculiar notions. But in that case would you please sneak into the public library some day when nobody is looking and ask for a standard textbook on physiology—*Howell's,* for example? It will tell you that salivary digestion (of cooked starch) begins in the mouth, if the food is properly masticated, and continues for half an hour to an hour after swallowing.

The old timers knew that the normal acidity of the gastric juices destroys ptyalin, the starch-digesting enzyme in the saliva, and so thought it didn't matter much whether one chewed thoroughly or gulped food down. Today we know, or should know, better. Insalivated by proper chewing, food remains in the fundic (upper) end of the stomach untouched by acid gastric juices for an hour or more while the digestion of starch continues—always provided a person has taken the time to masticate properly. If you cannot afford to do this—either because of inordinate hurry or on account of bad teeth or dentures—the symptoms that will develop will be legion. Your only consolation, dubious at best, is that millions of other Yankees will be in the same boat with you.

One of the things I remember about Saint Lutie is that she saw to it that I brushed my teeth at least once a day as part of my morning toilet. Since she lived at our house, two doors away from the schoolhouse, this was easily possible. I'm sure Miss Berner did what she did with the best intentions. Even today some people with no apparent interest in the manufacture and sale of dentifrices or toothbrushes not only brush their teeth regularly but use every conceivable stratagem to regularize the tooth-brushing habit, including ridiculous toothbrush drills in primary school.

Then, too, many dentists are still inspired by the slogan which made toothpaste big business, "A clean tooth never decays." This despite the fact that Americans, who wallow in tooth paste and brandish their toothbrushes in the eyes of "underprivileged" people, admittedly have the rottenest teeth in the world, with the possible exception of the English.

In impressive contrast with our namby-pamby oral or dental hygiene, the inhabitants of Tristan da Cunha, the "lonely isles" in the middle of the south Atlantic, have—or perhaps I should say still had when I was there in 1950—the finest teeth in all the world; and they had no use for toothbrushes or tooth pastes.

Prior to 1950 the islanders lived on undenaturized food: such vegetables as they could raise, seabirds' eggs, fish, crayfish or "rock lobster" which abound in the waters of the region, and occasionally fresh beef or mutton. Potatoes constituted the mainstay of their diet. But in 1949-1950 came a radical change. A London-Capetown company established a plant on the island for freezing or canning the crayfish to market in South America, the United States, England and South Africa. The company set up a store where the blessings(?) of civilization were made available to the inhabitants —refined white flour, refined white sugar, candy, syrup, namby-pamby "breakfast foods," even pop. By now, I have no doubt, the ship that brings supplies from Capetown and takes back the canned or frozen crayfish each month also brings a dentist from time to time to take care of the worsening teeth of the native inhabitants.

Chemical analysis of the drinking water on Tristan da Cunha showed it contained from one part fluorine in two million to one part in five million—the water comes from volcanic lakes high up above the plateau where the people live. Nutrition and health authorities generally consider one part of fluorine in a million parts of drinking water most desirable to prevent decay of the teeth.

Thanks to Saint Lutie's tuition I went on brushing my teeth nearly every day for about forty years. Then I quit wasting time and money on the silly practice. Since I came to my senses I have depended on (a) Diamond flat white birch toothpicks and (b) Ivory soap and water mouthwash to keep my teeth clean. This, I'm sure, has done as much to save my teeth as any amount of brushing with the most extravagant dentifrice (actually glorified soap) could have done. Keeping the teeth clean is merely a cosmetic matter anyway. The cleanest looking teeth may be badly decayed, while teeth that look dirty may be remarkably free from cavities. The condition of the teeth depends on the state of nutrition, and it seems to me that we Americans have proved abundantly that no matter how much we brush our teeth or what dentifrices we prefer, we can't save 'em on our ultrarefined, everyday American diet. We've been trying it for the better part of a century and our teeth are worse than ever. Hadn't we better try some other approach before they decay beyond restoration? My suggestion is better nutrition.

I have been trying to teach better nutrition through my syndicated health column for years, but this has become increasingly
difficult, if not altogether impossible, because it is as much as my
life—my newspaper life, that is—is worth to venture to specify
what I call "cheat-foods." Refined white flour, almost universally
used now instead of the real staff of life, tops my list. And when
the refined-white-flour people intimate that they prefer to advertise
in papers which do NOT carry Brady's column, out goes Brady's
column. You've no idea how many papers I have lost that way!
You might suppose I'd have more sense by now and would avoid
saying the things the barons object to and so prolong my life as a
teacher of health. But I'm afraid a column so censored would make
dreary reading. I'm sure it wouldn't be much fun writing it, and I
wonder how much real value it would have.

GOOD TEETH AND LONG LIFE   Years ago physicians, hy-
gienists and statisticians arrived at this general rule: for each inch
of girth over the average for age and height after thirty, deduct one
year—or is it two?—from the individual's life expectancy. Of
course there are exceptions—I said it was a general rule.

From long study and observation I arrived at a parallel rule for
teeth: For each tooth lost and not *immediately* replaced with a
functionally efficient artificial one—that is, one you can chew with
—deduct one to two years from your life expectancy. In other
words, the cost and value of a tooth is what you are willing to pay
for an extra year of life.

A young woman who lost several teeth in an accident was
awarded damages at the rate of $1000 per tooth in New England
in the 1940's—I regret I did not file the item telling of this adjudi-
cation. To me it did not seem excessive. Would you part with a
sound tooth or an efficient artificial one for $1000 unless you were
in the direst need of cash?

Fairly wide surveys indicate that more than fifty percent of the
population never do cut from one to all four wisdom teeth or third
molars. But even if a person past the middle period of life has only
four molars left, and all of his other twenty-four teeth (or dentures)
are functioning properly, he or she has a bonanza, the first of the

seven keys to V I T E. V I T E is seldom attainable without good dentistry. Your dentist is not merely a dispenser of good looks, but of functional efficiency, longevity—and VITE. Good teeth kept in good repair by regular prophylaxis, which is the detection and painless treatment of incipient caries or beginning cavities, will give you a paid-up insurance policy on youth.

According to U. S. Public Health Reports, 269 out of a thousand persons in rural, urban and metropolitan areas go to the dentist for such treatment once a year. The other 731 neglect their teeth or maybe brush like mad with glorified soap in the vain hope of preventing decay. They squander as much money that way as good dentistry or prophylaxis would cost and get nothing but grief for it in the end.

The survey also shows that most fillings are done for patients between fifteen and nineteen years of age. Frequency of fillings decreases steadily after that age. More extensive repairs, such as bridges and crowns, come in later life. Most extractions are at about the age of eight when temporary teeth are falling out and another peak comes between the ages of thirty-five and forty-five.

EAT FOR YOUR TEETH   Use of the jaws, gums and teeth as nature intended is another essential for the preservation of teeth.

In my judgment it is an excellent habit to chew some plain wheat every day, or some oats, or some barley, or some wild rice or some brown (unpolished) rice, and to eat some raw carrot, raw cabbage, raw turnip, raw potato, cucumber, radish, celery, tomato, lettuce, apple.

This does not imply, as some old-time dentists would have you think, that we must return to the habits of our remote ancestors and gnaw bones and eat only raw food. At that, it is a good plan to give the baby a bone to gnaw on as soon as he shows signs of cutting a tooth.

A certain amount of calcium (lime) and a certain amount of phosphorus is required to build good teeth. To insure metabolism, assimilation, utilization of this calcium and phosphorus, a certain amount of vitamin D is necessary to satisfy the demands of the expectant mother, the young infant, or the growing child. Some vitamin D supplement must be added to the daily ration: fish liver oil of one kind or another, or one of the synthetic viosterols such as condol in daily dose of ten or fifteen drops.

The body manufactures a certain amount of vitamin D itself if the naked skin is exposed to direct sunlight. Ultra-violet rays of sunlight convert sterols (fat-like substances) in the skin into vitamin D, which is carried in the circulation to the regions of the body where it is needed. So it is fair to say that the more the body is exposed to sunshine (short of sunburn) the better for the teeth.

Colored children sucking sugar cane in the sunny south are famous for their fine teeth. Their counterparts fed with sweetened condensed milk in the dark slums and hovels up north are exceedingly subject to rickets and defective teeth. The difference is sunshine vitamin D. Besides, sugar cane furnishes about three hundred times as much mineral matter, largely calcium and some phosphorus, as does refined sugar.

The vast majority of children coming to this country from southern Europe have sound teeth, whereas the vast majority of American children have defective ones. The children from Europe sometimes do not know what a toothbrush looks like until they enter American schools. At least this was true a generation ago. But who would broadcast such an observation over the radio or tell it to the world on the cover of a popular slick magazine?

I do not say it does the teeth or gums any harm to brush them if you like. I merely point out that the rite has nothing to do with prevention of decay. If there were any truth in the glib slogan that "a clean tooth never decays" it would follow that nobody has yet succeeded in getting his teeth quite clean by brushing them!

Day by day the weight of evidence increases to show that the conservation of the teeth, and their development, is a question of nutrition and the care of a good dentist. For that matter, from the standpoint of both healthy teeth and nutrition as a whole, a sound principle to follow is to include at least one fresh vegetable and one fresh fruit in every meal, or at any rate at dinnertime. It is also advisable to include a salad in every dinner. This should be made of raw—not cooked—vegetables or relishes and should be something to chew, something worth chewing for its palatability and appetizing value, as well as for the vitamins and minerals it contains.

Chewing is exercise. It also massages the gums. While I am no enthusiast for the rite of brushing, I do believe that vigorous massage of the gums three times a day is a must for preventing decay, and what better massage than that which comes with eating a raw apple, turnip, carrot or raw cabbage. I am also all for massage of the gums with the clean finger. For that matter, the only value of brushing, to my mind, is the casual massage the gums get during the process.

MOTHERS' AND BABIES' TEETH Modern dentistry recognizes that baby or milk teeth, although they are temporary, deserve proper care and preservation. Baby teeth should be filled in order to prevent premature loss, otherwise they will not have served their purpose of being a sound foundation for the development of strong, even teeth later on. Neglected cavities in baby teeth may also become the source of focal infection quite as serious as a septic mouth condition in an adult.

The nutrition of the mother during the prenatal period determines in large measure the character of her child's future teeth. It is, therefore, one of the essentials of the expectant mother's diet to receive an extra large daily ration of vitamin D, as well as adequate amounts of vitamins A and C. Eggs, fresh fruits, fresh vegetables and plenty of milk are a must, for if there is any shortage in the essential minerals or vitamins it is the mother who will suffer. For the fetus is a parasite and will rob her tissues of whatever it requires, which explains why pregnant women so frequently experience rapid decay of the teeth as well as other manifestations of undernutrition.

The enamel of the teeth is a natural armor against microorganisms or mouth acids or other theoretically harmful influences. The enamel is about 97 per cent lime phosphate. The main structure of the teeth, the dentine, is also composed principally of calcium, or lime, and phosphorus. So is the bone of the jaw.

These three elements are the ones most frequently deficient in the refined food of the average American family. But even if the diet does supply nearly or quite enough calcium and phosphorus to fulfill the requirements of the body, there may still be a fault in the assimilation, utilization and retention of these essential elements, which do not take place unless there is also sufficient vitamin D in the daily intake.

Getting an adequate daily ration of the sunshine vitamin is not so easy. Few foods suitable for human consumption contain enough of it for optimal nutrition. The only foods that contain it at all are fresh milk, cream and butter, egg yolk, oysters, fresh or canned salmon, fresh or canned sardines, a few other fish or shellfish and fish liver oil. On the whole, however, so far as is known, vitamin D is vitamin D, unit for unit, whether derived from food, oil, or from ultraviolet irradiation of ergosterol, a fat-like substance found in certain foods but chiefly in special strains of brewer's yeast.

The dentist who serves his patients well should, then, make it his business to see that they are properly instructed about these simple facts of optimal nutrition. This goes double for the parents of growing children. On the whole, sound dietary habits, as discussed in this chapter and in other chapters to follow, are good general insurance for sound teeth.

Chapter Three

TAKE CARE OF YOUR MOUTH

While many people realize, at least in theory, that periodic dental checkups are something they owe themselves, information about mouth troubles unrelated to toothache is alarmingly meager. Until recently, for instance, the general attitude toward pyorrhea was pure fatalism: if you got it you must just resign yourself to having all your teeth pulled. This of course was—and still may be—true when the condition is long neglected. Other oral disturbances may have even sadder results—but they needn't, if you are alert.

TRENCH MOUTH Fortunately Vincent's angina, or "trench mouth," is far less prevalent today than it was several years ago. People must have learned to avoid unnecessary exposure to the infection which is highly contagious and is communicated usually via eating and drinking utensils which haven't been properly sterilized by washing with hot water and soap, via unsterilized instruments—and via kissing. In the course of a local epidemic it was suggested that all dentists, even when sore mouth was not evident, should give treatment with sodium perborate before and after dental treatment. Such treatment, once a day, with sodium perborate made into a thin paste with water and spread over all the teeth and gums, especially over any red or raw areas on gums, tongue, lips or inside cheeks, held in the mouth for five minutes and then rinsed out with warm water, is usually all that is necessary to clear up the condition. But if the mouth doesn't respond promptly, it is a good plan to consult a reputable doctor or dentist. For the mouth sores of "trench mouth" are sometimes confused with smoker's patches, galvanic sore mouth, simple canker sores or ulceration from jagged or broken teeth. They may also be confused with incipient cancer or the primary sort (chancre) or the secondary sores (mucus patches) of syphilis. Wrong diagnosis— often self-diagnosis—may cause much needless worry and fear, but on the other hand in the exceptional case may create a sense of false security.

GALVANIC SORE MOUTH   It seems to be the ill luck of a small number of those who have two dissimilar metals in the mouth to suffer from painful ulcers of the cheek or the tongue mucous membrane, ulcers which heal but poorly and soon reappear. Why only a few patients with, say, gold and copper alloys plus silver or amalgam in various fillings, inlays, crowns, bridges and the like, suffer from these painful ulcers, please do not ask me. Possibly the saliva of some persons is a better electrolyte than is the saliva of others, and makes a more efficient miniature galvanic battery by its action on the dissimilar metals. Anyway, normal saliva is a fair electrolyte—it need not be particularly acid; nor does the use of alkaline mouthwash seem to alleviate or correct the trouble in these cases.

Galvanic ulcers may be mistaken for obstinate "canker sores" which they resemble to a degree; the galvanic sores do not heal as readily as canker sores, however, and usually the galvanic ulcers are directly opposite or in the path between the dentures which are responsible. In some cases galvanic sore mouth is mistaken for smoker's patches, medically called leucoplakia.

In any case of galvanic sore mouth the practical question arises, whether to remove the gold or the amalgam fillings. One or the other metal must be removed and replaced with a metal similar to that present in the mouth. In some cases it is more practical to remove the recently installed gold and substitute for it one of the same metal as that composing the fillings present in the teeth. In other cases the amalgam fillings should be removed, replaced with gold like that of the crown, bridge or inlay already installed.

CANKER SORES   Grandma used to say that swearing or naughty words brought canker sores, so I always confined my incidental remarks to "gracious" and "oh" until I had my first crop of canker sores and then I cut loose, but it didn't help any, that I could notice.

That we docs haven't the slightest idea what causes canker sores is manifest to the discerning reader when we call canker sore "aphthous stomatitis"—stomatitis being atrocious medical Latin-Greek for inflammation of the mouth, and aphtha being Greek for ulcer.

From what I can learn of the general medical view, canker sores are more likely to occur on a basis of malnutrition or nutritional deficiency, perhaps inadequate daily intake of vitamins essential for the most healthy state of the mucous membrane. The direct or precipitating cause may be slight injury of the membrane by accidental biting, by a rough or jagged tooth, by the toothbrush, by excessively hot food or drink or a sharp crust or bit of bone in the food. There is also a theory that canker sores may depend on focal infection in some cases, as for example, a septic focus in the tonsil.

Admitting that doctors know nothing about the cause of canker sores, they may still cure them by treatment . . . If you are subject to them you should take special pains to have any septic focus about your teeth, gums or tonsils cleared up. You should see to it that you get adequate vitamins daily. You should make sure the sores are neither smoker's patch, galvanic sore mouth nor "trench mouth." Above all, do not put off consulting the physician about any persistent sores on the lip or tongue or in the throat in the comfortable belief that they are just "cold" sores.

Gently rinsing the mouth a dozen times a day with lukewarm solution of a heaping teaspoonful of boric acid dissolved in a pint of water, especially before and after eating, will help ordinary canker sores. Gently touching each sore once a day with a wisp of cotton on the end of a toothpick moistened with equal parts of glycerine and tincture of iodine smarts momentarily but seems to relieve the soreness.

Recently laboratory investigators have observed that vitamin C promotes the natural healing process in ulcer, wound or burn. Today comes a letter from a reader who suggests the following treat-

ment for canker sores which she says has worked satisfactorily for
two members of her own family:

> Place a piece of lemon on the sore part and keep it there for 20
> minutes. The sores will cease to annoy and disappear within a few
> hours.

Lemon juice is of course rich in vitamin C. All I know about
the lemon treatment is that it can do no harm. I leave it to the
reader to determine whether it does any good.

WHITE PATCHES IN THE MOUTH Leucoplakia or leuko-
plakia is the medical term for white patches on the tongue, inner
surface of the cheek or sometimes about the genitals of either sex.
The thickened, whitish patches, accompanied with some local irritation and perhaps increased sensitivity to heat or other stimulation, are generally painless and cause only a stiffness of the affected
part. This stiffness or lack of normal flexibility or pliability ultimately leads to fissuring and in the course of years ulceration and
finally malignancy (cancerous degeneration) may occur.

These white patches are obstinate and difficult to heal. They
are sometimes called "smoker's patches," and it may be true that
they are found most frequently in smokers, but certainly leucoplakia does occur in persons who have never smoked at all.

We don't know what causes it. But we do know that one with
leucoplakia must absolutely stop using tobacco, have any rough
teeth or fillings attended to by the dentist, and in long standing
cases submit to one or another destructive treatment of the patch
—carbon dioxide freezing, electro-coagulation, actual cautery or
radium treatments in the hands of a doctor skilled in such work.

The penalty of neglect of proper treatment of leucoplakia is in
too many cases—

Cancer of tongue, cheek or mouth. When cancerous degeneration begins in a white patch the lesion usually but not always becomes somewhat painful, and swollen "glands" (lymph nodes) or
kernels may be felt under the jaw or in the side of the neck; the
white patch becomes reddish, velvety or raw looking.

CANCER FROM NEGLECTED TEETH Cancer more commonly
occurs in the mouth as a consequence of prolonged slight irrita-

tion by a jagged or broken tooth or a rough or broken denture, without any sign of white patch.

Pipe smoking is well known as an exciting factor of cancer of the lip. Cigar smoking has been regarded as an exciting factor of cancer of the throat. Cigarette smoking seems more frequently associated with cancer of the tongue—whether from slight but constant irritation or just because so many out of the whole population are smokers.

At any rate good dentistry has a definite prophylactic value, helps to prevent cancer; whereas cheap bargain dentistry by the type of practitioner who can't gain and hold a living practice in the ethical way—through the good will of his satisfied patients—must be reckoned one of the predisposing causes of cancer in the mouth.

STAINS ON THE TEETH In some regions where the drinking water contains fluorine in sufficient quantity (more than one part per million) children from six to eighteen years of age show peculiar staining of teeth—black, brown or yellow, or sometimes ghastly opaque white spots in the enamel. This may be prevented only by providing drinking water comparatively free from fluorides. No method of removing fluoride from water has as yet been found. The stain cannot be removed, once it develops.

Green stains which are not removed by brushing with soap, ordinary dentifrice, soda, willow charcoal or salt, may be cleared away by brushing with a drop or two of tincture of iodine (*no more*) on the wet brush, followed by brushing with a few drops of aromatic spirits of ammonia on the wet brush.

Mere dark or yellowish discoloration of the teeth is best removed by frequent rinsing of the mouth with weak hydrogen peroxide solution (teaspoonful of standard peroxide with five or six spoonfuls of water). Or by brushing the teeth from time to time with sodium perborate powder or with one of the sweetened and aromatically flavored preparations of sodium perborate designed as mouthwash.

The application of the iodine and ammonia as above described may be repeated several days in succession, or as often as twice a week for a child, or every day for an adult.

When tartar deposits discolor the teeth, only the dentist may remove them without risk of injuring the enamel.

There is no objection to the use of wooden toothpicks for keeping the spaces between the teeth free from food detritus—in fact good dentists advise this. Metal toothpicks should not be used.

As a general rule when one or more teeth become darkened to a noticeable degree it is wisest to submit to one's dentist the question of attempting to bleach or brighten them.

A so-called "dead" tooth usually appears darker or more opaque than a normal tooth. Such a tooth is not "dead" but pulpless. It may still serve a useful purpose in the jaw for many years. Some dentists radically condemn pulpless teeth because they are more likely to be infected about the roots than are normal teeth. There is time enough to consider extracting a tooth when we have definite evidence that the root is infected or the source of a focal infection which is accountable for some systematic trouble. Doctors or dentists who urge extraction of a useful or apparently sound tooth on X-ray evidence alone, or on the principle that a pulpless tooth may some day become a source of trouble, are not practicing medicine but a kind of quackery.

THE CAUSE AND CURE OF PYORRHEA   Most physicians and dentists now accept the view that pyorrhea is a manifestation of faulty nutrition, and full co-operation between physician and dentist is necessary to check the progress of the trouble.

Lest the casual reader get a wrong impression, I beg to explain again that nutrition means much more than proper food or diet. It means rather the digestion, assimilation and utilization of food, water and oxygen to build up and repair body tissues and to liberate energy to do the work of the body. The clothing one wears or discards, the exercise one gets daily or avoids, and the sunshine one cultivates or dodges may be as important factors as the kind of food one eats, in the causation or prevention of pyorrhea.

There is considerable clinical and scientific evidence that insufficient vitamin C in the daily intake is one factor of excessive caries or decay of teeth and of pyorrhea, just as it is in scurvy. Pyorrhea is defined as suppurative inflammation of the periosteum or bone-covering membrane lining the tooth sockets, with shrink-age or atrophy of the gums and loosening of the teeth. Gingivitis is inflammation of the gums. Both are essentially the same de-generative disease and, according to modern authorities, the con-dition variously called pyorrhea alveolaris, Riggs' disease, chronic gingivitis and Fauchard's disease, is fundamentally a manifestation of faulty nutrition.

We can offer only general information and advice concerning causes, prevention and relief. It remains for your own dentist to treat specific conditions in your case. He knows best whether your teeth require, for instance, scaling to remove tartar or calcareous deposits or perhaps other prophylactic measures to maintain as nearly as possible normal function. Remember, regular, normal use is the best prevention against atrophy, shrinkage or wasting of tissues.

With respect to the conservation of the teeth, people too often forget that non-use, whether of some of the teeth on one side or of all of the teeth, inevitably leads to weakening, wasting or atrophy. Critical inspection of the mouth of the pyorrhea patient usually shows plainly that the patient, in earlier years, has neglected to have necessary dental treatment and repairs, or has indulged in the false economy of makeshift work by dental quacks or cheap-johns.

One who has any trouble with a tooth can make no better in-vestment than the services of a dentist whose skill may save that tooth. An individual who appreciates the value of health and phys-ical efficiency will never hesitate to spend a week's income on the effort to save or restore the damaged or decayed tooth. On the other hand any fool can and probably will conclude at once that extraction of the troublesome tooth is the right solution. Today you can buy a fine set of teeth for a thousand dollars, but not for a thousand dollars a tooth can you buy 'em as good as your own were before you allowed them to fall into dis-use and dis-ease.

The principal nutritional deficiencies which competent investi-gators consider factors of pyorrhea are (1) diet poor in calcium and phosphorus, (2) too little food requiring chewing, (3) lack of vitamin A which is important especially in the development of the soft tissues about the teeth, (4) lack of vitamin C and

(5) lack of vitamin D, the sunlight vitamin, essential for proper utilization of calcium and phosphorus. Some doctors also believe that neglect of or improper technique in brushing teeth is a contributing factor.

When your dentist extracts a tooth or teeth and advises filling the gap with a bridge, there are more important considerations than personal appearance which should guide you in making a decision. Functionally efficient teeth—a full set of 'em—help maintain good mastication, and this in turn helps maintain good nutrition of gums and teeth and prevent the encroachment of pyorrhea and the progress of caries. Finally, proper daily use of all the teeth favors the ideal state of nutrition necessary for general physical fitness, good spirits—in short, for V I T E.

THE FOCAL PRINCIPLE   It is neither a theory nor a fad, but a well established principle of practice that certain systemic ailments such as arthritis, neuritis, valvular heart disease, perhaps some cases of peptic ulcer, are caused by focal infection. That is to say the joint, nerve, heart valve or lining of stomach or duodenum becomes inflamed from lodgment therein of germs carried through the blood stream from a nidus or focus elsewhere in the body, in the tonsils, about the teeth or gums, in root canal, where the germs have gained a foothold and multiplied for weeks, months or years before the more or less accidental embolism or travelling of a colony or clump of the germs through the bloodstream to the place of lodgment occurs. Strains of the notorious Streptococcus are most frequently concerned in focal infection, especially Streptococcus hemolyticus (blood destroying) and Streptococcus viridans (green colonies).

Indiscriminate application of the focal infection principle in practice has brought it into low repute. Certainly many sound teeth have been needlessly sacrificed in a blind hope of "getting rid of the poison." On the other hand, "regrets over the late discovery of a septic focus heretofore overlooked or ignored" are even greater in some instances than those over the unavailing sacrifice of useful teeth.

It is a matter of the best judgment of doctor and dentist, after consultation in the individual case, whether to attempt to eradicate a presumptive focus when this means removal of a useful tooth. Further than to say that it is always a question of opinion whether an infected tooth is actually the focus, I leave the problem there.

The test of the principle, the only test, is the result of the removal of the focus. Not the immediate result merely; in some cases the immediate reaction is apparently aggravation of the joint trouble or whatever the condition may be; but the ultimate result of such treatment becomes manifest generally several weeks, perhaps two or three months after the extraction or other operation.

In case several teeth are infected and doctor and dentist agree upon the advisability of removing them, it is usually wise, in the presence of systemic trouble of any considerable severity, to carry out the extractions in several sittings at intervals of several weeks, and not to remove more than two teeth at any one time. In this way the patient suffers no overwhelming septic flood, but rather gets the benefit of a moderate or therapeutic dose of autogenous bacterin or bacterial "vaccine," the bacteria or their products absorbed from the fresh wound area.

As I mention above, so-called "dead" teeth, properly called pulpless, but not dead as long as the tooth structure gets any nourishment—a controversial point among modern dental pathologists —have so commonly been inculpated and circumstantially proved responsible for focal infection, even though the patient is not aware of any trouble in the tooth, that many good dentists, not all, urge extraction of such teeth as the safest course in any case. If I had a pulpless tooth serving a useful purpose in my mouth I'd want more than the mere knowledge of its presence or even an equivocal X-ray shadow around the root, to convince me to sacrifice the tooth. On the other hand, if I were developing some vague chronic joint condition not otherwise accounted for, I'd gamble the tooth against the chance of arresting the progress of the joint trouble. And remember, I consider every functionally efficient tooth, real or artificial, worth one hundred thousand cents.

Chapter Four

DON'T CHEAT YOURSELF
OF VITAMINS

Until 1926 it was generally believed that "vitamin B" was a single entity. In that year Smith and Hendrick showed that it consisted of two factors, vitamin B_1, later known as thiamin, and vitamin B_2 or G, later called riboflavin. Since 1926 a raft of vitamins have been split off from the original Vitamin B. Some of these are pantothenic acid, pyrodoxin, niacin or nicotinic acid, folic acid, biotin, B_{12}. So it is now customary to refer to vitamin B in food as vitamin B complex. To try to tell more about the factors, the vitamins that compose natural vitamin B complex, would be pointless and confusing.

It is enough to say that the richest natural food source of vitamin B complex, especially vitamin B_1 or thiamin, is *plain wheat,* or the grain as it comes from the thresher. And the richest natural food source of vitamin B_2, G or riboflavin, is milk and its derivative, cheese.

Milk, provided it is fresh, raw, certified milk, is also the best source of vitamins A and D, which are contained in the cream or butter fat.

It therefore follows that bread and milk, or bread and cheese, make the most satisfactory snack, lunch or even full meal for child and adult. But again let me stress that the milk must be raw, from tuberculin-tested and certified herds, and the bread made of whole wheat, freshly ground and not doctored or "refined" in any way. Raw milk from cows on pasture even supplies vitamin C.

By "most satisfactory" I mean nutritionally most adequate.

Prior to the fourth decade of the twentieth century, physicians had little knowledge of the science of nutrition. Indeed this whole science is barely 40 years old, founded, it is fair to say, by Prof. Henry C. Sherman of Columbia University (*Chemistry of Food and Nutrition*) and Prof. Elmer V. McCollum of Johns Hopkins University (*The Newer Knowledge of Nutrition*) in the '30's.

Away back when I was an honest family doctor—and that, we submit, must have been a long while ago if ever—we used many words we didn't quite understand. But this hardly mattered, for our patients did not see through us. Words such as malnutrition, trophic, dystrophic, well-nourished had little meaning for them or for us.

Trophia or trophic means nourishment or nourished. Atrophy means undernourishment, lack of nutrition or wasting away. Hypertrophy means the state of being overnourished, enlargement, or overgrowth.

In an attempt to explain what we ourselves did not know, some medical sage conceived the notion of "trophic" nerves. These were supposed to be elusive nervelets resembling capillary blood vessels. You couldn't see 'em and nobody had ever isolated one, not even under the microscope, but you had better believe they existed or the big boys in the medical profession wouldn't like you very well.

"Well nourished" meant well fed. "Malnutrition" meant that some poor soul wasn't getting enough to eat.

Another term we used learnedly, if loosely, was "well balanced diet." Just what we meant by it I was never quite sure, but again it made no difference for the customers never asked—they didn't want to seem dumb. Some doctors still use this device of obfuscation to cover their ignorance of nutrition, a well balanced diet being something like "the common cold" and "chronic arthritis." You do not ask the doctor to tell you just what it is, for any darned fool is supposed to know . . .

When a patient asks whether it is necessary or advisable to supplement the everyday ultrarefined diet with extra vitamins and/or minerals, the doctor is still quite likely to say that if one follows a reasonably varied diet of meat, fish, eggs, milk, fruit, vegetables and cereals, one will get all the vitamins and minerals one needs from everyday food.

This is not altogether true in view of our present practice of first emasculating, then doctoring such foods as refined white flour with vitamins and minerals, irradiating milk with vitamin D, margarine with vitamin A and so forth. Although this practice is widely sanctioned by medical and health authorities, the truth is that anyone following the standard diet of most middle class Americans today is almost certain to suffer in one way or another from insufficient intake of essential vitamins and minerals unless he or she regularly supplements this diet.

Indeed, it is my conviction that most of the minor complaints, for which people are prone to dose themselves with plain or fancy nostrums, are really manifestations of nutritional deficiencies and so will not respond to any kind of medication. Please don't misinterpret my teaching, though—I only say *most minor complaints* are of this nature.

In my judgment the most widespread vitamin deficiency in America is B complex deficiency. And the most widespread mineral shortage is either iodine or calcium deficiency.

The B complex shortage is due mainly to our huge consumption of refined white flour as a staple of everyday diet. It is from this refined white flour and from refined white sugar that most Americans get the bulk of their daily calories. But in the refining of wheat, which is the richest source of vitamin B complex, nearly *all* the vitamins—B complex, A and E—are removed along with the bran or outer coat and the germ or heart of the kernel. Little is left in the flour except starch.

Whole wheat flour begins to turn rancid in a matter of days, whereas refined white flour keeps indefinitely. This explains why whole wheat flour is not marketable at appreciable distances from the mill or at appreciable intervals of time after the milling.

Unfortunately consumers in this country have been conveniently taught to prefer refined white flour. They now consider it "purer" than plain wheat flour. They also have been told it is more easily digested.

This is what Robert R. Williams, Sc.D., distinguished nutrition authority, has to say on the millers' practice of discarding wheat germ: "Man commits a crime against nature when he eats the starch from the seed and throws away the mechanism necessary for the metabolism of that starch."

Experimental evidence seems to indicate that it is the thiamin, or B_1, and the riboflavin, or B_2, in the B complex that are "necessary for the metabolism of starch." Numerous persons with diabetes have reported to me that when they supplement their diet with a good daily ration of vitamin B complex they require less insulin. I must admit, however, that Dr. Elliott P. Joslin, top authority on diabetes, tells me, and states in his book, that he has not observed any such effect from vitamin B complex.

Commenting on the attitude of Americans toward the staff of life a Kansas reader once told me: "We live surrounded by miles and miles of wheat fields. We make our living growing wheat. Yet it remained for you to teach us how good it is to eat. Now even the children prefer it to 'namby-pamby' breakfast foods."

This woman, like her parents and grandparents, had been inculcated by the cheat-food barons with the notion that plain wheat is not fit for human consumption until it has been "processed" and packed in pretty packages. It is a commentary on American credulity that so many wheat farmers do not know what plain wheat tastes like.

Come to think of it, the Brady family on Chapel Street in Canandiagua was probably the poorest in Ontario County in the Gay Nineties, with seven and sometimes eight of us living on $30 to $35 a month, supplemented by the vegetables, fruit, milk, eggs, butter, greens and meat we raised in our own garden and from working rich people's land on shares. Yet we lived well. Still, I remember we spent a considerable amount of cash money for a barrel of refined white flour every little while. Too bad there was no Ol' Doc Brady around at the time to wise us up about plain wheat. We did, after all, have a coffee mill!

I still recall with pleasure how good wheat was to chew—it worked into something as good as store gum.

WHAT TO EAT   As I keep saying, popular prejudices against the use of plain wheat as a staple and mainstay of diet are cultivated by commercial interests and have no foundation in physiology. Certain invalids may not be able to digest plain wheat, but actual tests have proved that normally people do digest it perfectly and thrive on it. I believe a good many common ailments could be avoided if we would set up in every kitchen a wheat bin and a suitable mill or grinder for preparing meal and flour as needed.

In the process of refining white flour other essentials are removed from the wheat besides the vitamin B complex, E and A. Milling and refining also removes four-fifths of the iron, nearly four-fifths of the phosphorus and nearly one-half of the calcium, or lime, in the wheat. The finished product yields what some nutritionists have called empty calories—it is totally inadequate as a well-rounded food.

Some old time physicians seem to go along with the notion about the indigestibility of the outer part of the kernel, or bran. Yet actual physiological observation, notably by Hindhede, has proven that not only is it well digested by the human stomach but that bread made of whole wheat sustains health and efficiency, both of which become impaired if the bread in the diet is changed to white bread. Finally, just as from years or perhaps even a lifetime of habit people develop a preference for white bread, so this factor of taste easily adjusts itself when they discover how zestful and appetizing are the breads, cakes and other dishes in which whole wheat is the main ingredient.

Since most fruits and vegetables contain some vitamin B it is possible to get enough of it to maintain optimal health from a well balanced diet alone. But once refined white flour is used, the diet is likely to be deficient in vitamin B in proportion to the extent to which white flour is used instead of the entire wheat.

More than half of the calories in the average American diet today are derived from foods which supply only about $\frac{1}{6}$ of a milligram of vitamin B daily. In 1840 the average American diet supplied in the foods containing or yielding the same number of calories (whole wheat flour ground in the stone mill, other whole grain or cereal foods, crude brown sugar, molasses) probably 2 mg. of Vitamin B_1 (thiamin) daily.

One and one half mg. of Vitamin B_1, together with the other B complex factors that naturally occur with B_1, probably more nearly represents the daily ration of vitamin B complex required to maintain functional efficiency and health. The average American diet today supplies perhaps ⅓ milligram of B_1 and a proportionate deficiency of the other B complex factors, not to mention the other vitamins essential for vigorous health.

Theoretically, it might be possible to get an adequate daily ration of the essential vitamins and minerals by greater use of the "protective" foods—particularly milk, green vegetables and fruits. But in practice, in order to secure the vitamin B_1 which has been lost during the past century as a result of refinement in milling of wheat, one would have to consume tremendous and impossible quantities of these "protective" foods—something like one and a quarter pounds of fruit, one and a quarter pounds of potatoes, one and a half pounds of other vegetables and five pints of milk every day!

In order to get an adequate amount of Vitamin B_1 as it occurs in the B complex, one would have to eat not less than nine ounces of plain wheat in one form or another; or about four ounces of fresh wheat germ; or one or two B-Nutron tablets (Nion), or a teaspoonful or two of B-Nutron Syrup daily.

It is easy to eat plain wheat in one form or another, provided it is served in a variety of dishes or recipes which appeal to the taste. It is not so easy to eat wheat germ every day in anything like the quantity mentioned. But even if you can't eat enough of it, you may still derive considerable benefit from daily consumption of whatever amount of these vitamin B complex rich foods you can contrive to include in your diet. And if you keep a supply of Nion tablets or syrup on hand it is a simple matter to eat enough of them to make sure you will get an optimal ration of vitamin B complex, that is, more than just enough to prevent deficiency manifestations, enough to maintain better-than-average functional efficiency, or what I call VITE.

Wheat germ is best purchased at the mill, any mill where they will bother to catch out some when a customer calls for it. Such wheat germ is fresh, most palatable, high in vitamin E as well as B complex. It begins to lose potency after a week or two. So buy only enough at a time to last you for one or two weeks—usually two pounds is sufficient. Some food stores and some large drug-stores handle it, but the wheat germ one buys at the mill is in my opinion best, regardless of the imposing packaging and the imposing language you get with the fancy-priced store-bought goods. Some mills ship wheat germ by parcel post on order if customers prefer to buy a few pounds at a time. I cannot undertake to specify mills or their terms—drop a postcard with return card to any mill in your vicinity and inquire about it.

The cheapness of wheat as a staple in the diet is an important consideration. Some one has called milk "the most nearly perfect food." For the infant it may be, but for the growing child and the adult, wheat is even more adequate. There can also be no question but that plain wheat, as bought from farmer, mill, feed or seed store and ground and cooked at home, is the most economical of foods. Wheat contains approximately 14 per cent of protein, two point seven per cent of fat and 75 per cent of carbohydrate, compared with milk which contains three point five per cent protein, four per cent fat, and five per cent carbohydrate. Less than 12 per cent of wheat is water; more than 85 per cent of milk is water.

One English mother raised some of the healthiest children you could wish to see on daily rations of plain wheat which was allowed to soak for one hour or more in hot milk, but not boiled.

An American father finds the following dish "the finest breakfast food in the world": Put such quantity of wheat as desired (not too much, for it swells in cooking) in water and boil for five minutes. Then let it stand from 12 to 24 hours. After this long soaking boil on moderate fire till soft as desired. (The preliminary boiling is to prevent fermentation.) Keep it in the refrigerator box and heat up as required.

An American housewife writes, "We steam our wheat for cereal, and the leftovers are stored in the refrigerator. Then I add this cooked wheat to waffles, muffins, etc., usually adding one to one and a half cupfuls in place of the white flour in the recipe, and perhaps increase the amount of egg. We steam the wheat in an aluminum pan. It cooks thoroughly in an hour and is fluffy, with separate grains, not gummy.

A Milwaukee man says: I bought a bushel of wheat at the mill, cleaned and ready to grind. Here's how to make pancakes warranted to get you up early in the morning: Beat one egg thoroughly, add salt to taste and one tablespoonful sugar. Add a pint of sour milk in which a teaspoonful of soda has been dissolved. Thicken to batter consistency with finely ground wheat, beat well and cook in well greased griddle or skillet. We find the ordinary coffee mill adjusted to grind fine a satisfactory wheat grinder.

Here is Ol' Doc Brady's own recipe for wheat gems: Mix a tablespoonful old-fashioned molasses (no sulphur in it), a cupful of sweet milk, two cupfuls finely ground wheat, a pinch of salt, two tablespoonfuls melted butter, one egg thoroughly beaten; finally stir in a teaspoonful of baking powder. Bake in gem tins.

A Connecticut man says plain wheat porridge for breakfast beats all the "sawdust" cereals and is much cheaper: "We grind the wheat as fine as possible in a coffee mill, place in double boiler, cook for 15 or 20 minutes the night before, set on back of stove and next morning place over heat just long enough to heat through.

Hardware dealers have hand grist mills which are convenient for grinding not only wheat but rye, corn, peanuts, soy beans and other grains. Every well managed household should have such a mill.

An Oregon judge contributes this recipe for wheat cookies: Two cupfuls finely ground wheat; half cupful molasses; two tablespoonfuls butter or lard; one egg; two teaspoonfuls baking powder; half cupful milk. Beat together butter, egg, milk and molasses, stir in the other ingredients. Drop mixed batter with spoon onto greased tins and bake half an hour in hot oven.

An Iowa editor calls the macaroons he nibbles as he reads "muncharoons." His recipe is five or six tablespoonfuls coarsely ground wheat, a cupful chopped almonds, one egg, half a cupful unsulphured molasses. Beat egg and molasses, add the wheat and nuts and bake on buttered tins in medium oven twenty minutes.

It remains for a Minnesota cook to furnish the recipe for Plain Wheat Bread:

Scald one and a half cupfuls milk and cool to blood temperature. Make a smooth paste of one tablespoonful molasses, three tablespoonfuls lard, one and a half cakes compressed yeast and half cupful lukewarm water and add the milk. Then add six cupfuls well ground wheat meal to make a sponge. Beat the sponge five minutes, cover and set in warm place till it rises to double size. Now add one teaspoonful salt and, if desired, half cupful raisins or half to one cupful finely chopped walnut meats. Beat again five minutes in bowl. Half fill greased tins with dough and rub dough lightly with lard. Let stand in warm place till dough in tins rises to double size. Then bake for about an hour. Take pains to avoid jarring dough when putting in oven, lest it fall flat. If you add raisins you should first soak them for ten minutes in scalding water, then dry.

In incorporating plain wheat in any recipe, do not worry about digestion if the taste of the dish is pleasing. It is certain that anyone who can digest any wheat product cooked, can digest plain wheat raw or only slightly cooked. In fact many people prefer wheat not too thoroughly cooked. The unchanged starch in undercooked wheat serves a wholesome, healthful purpose—it favors a vigorous growth of lactic bacilli in the intestinal tract which promotes normal digestion and opposes putrefaction.

In recent years, according to federal statistics, the per capita consumption of wheat has gradually declined while the per capita consumption of sugar has gradually increased. For health's sake this is not as it should be.

Lay in a peck or a bushel of wheat and see for yourself how good it is to eat.

Hand power or electric power mills for household use may be obtained from The Straub Co., 4059 Ridge Ave., Philadelphia 29, Pa., or from Landers, Frary & Clark, New Britain, Conn. These will grind wheat into flour. You may also dig up grandmother's coffee mill.

THE MYSTERY OF VITAMIN E   From certain popular magazine articles and periodic "scientific" abstracts, emanating mainly from an institution in Canada and concerning vitamin E one might very well get the impression that this vitamin works like magic. Especially is this true if one hasn't time to study the question thoroughly or if one is not qualified to judge.

Wheat germ and green leafy vegetables, especially lettuce, are the richest sources of vitamin E. There is good reason to believe that the average American diet supplies very little vitamin E. A vitamin E deficiency *may* be a factor of *sterility*. As for prevention or treatment of heart disease, there seems to be only conjectural ground for the use of vitamin E.

Still a third "indication" for the use of vitamin E is muscular dystrophy, multiple sclerosis, progressive muscular atrophy etc. I am sorry to say that in my opinion there is insufficient evidence to show that vitamin E has any special remedial value in these cases. However it can do no harm to try it for a month or two.

Wheat germ oil is virtually vitamin E and nothing else—undoubtedly the best method of taking it in. But it is difficult to understand why wheat germ oil should ever be taken in preference to whole wheat germ, as Bicknell and Prescott's *The Vitamins in Medicine* points out. Certainly, the oil cannot contain anything not present in the parent germ and it is equally certain that much of value may be lost in preparation—the vitamin B complex and minerals, for instance. And I for one beg to carry the argument one step further and point out that certainly, the wheat germ cannot contain anything not present in plain wheat.

So now I call for my pipe and head for the bowling green, wondering whether the preponderance of emasculated food in our diet may not account for the relatively high incidence of sterility in American men and women today.

Chapter Five

YOU'VE GOT TO HAVE CALCIUM

The body of a healthy adult weighing 150 pounds contains two and a quarter pounds of calcium, or lime. This quantity is essential to give a person the attributes variously known as vigor, vitality, backbone, perseverance, nerve, fortitude, stamina, will power, guts, determination, grit, elasticity, courage and self-confidence. That an adult's body must contain that amount of calcium is a scientific fact which no chemist, physiologist or physician will deny. That calcium controls "backbone," courage and other such qualities is just one of Brady's vagaries, as the fancy specialists and "clinic" boys characterize my teachings when patients venture to inquire. It is only fair to warn you that the merchants of medicine call me "Old Calcium Brady."

I suppose, like anyone else who's lost some of his marbles, I would be the last to recognize such a thing. But if I am nutty, I come by it naturally: My father had a wonderful streak of lunacy in him which I remember with affection and delight.

For instance, when I was a freshman medical student, father's current insanity was sand eating. He kept on hand a box of white sand, washed and baked, and took a teaspoonful once or twice daily—to promote good stomach and bowel function, he said. He urged me to do likewise, but I couldn't bring myself to down a single spoonful. Father's argument was that if sand and gravel were good for birds and mammals, they should be good for human beings. I must say he seemed to thrive on it for years. Ultimately he did succumb to cancer of the intestine, but whether his sand eating contributed to this I do not know.

My belief in the nutritional value of calcium and its value to general well being has a better foundation than my father's trust in sand, for I arrived at it through long years of study of physiology, nutrition, therapeutics and pathology. "Mairsy dotes "n" dozy dotes" has nothing to do with it. I am, however, permanently impressed by the dictum of one of the founders of the science of nutrition, Henry C. Sherman, who writes, "The ordinary mixed diet of Americans and Europeans, at least among dwellers in cities and towns, is probably more often deficient in calcium than in any other chemical element."

In his famous textbook, *Chemistry of Food and Nutrition,* he further states: "In adults there may be a long-continued loss of calcium without the appearance of symptoms because the losses from the blood and soft tissues may be replaced by calcium withdrawn from the bones."

As I mention in the chapters on teeth, the calcium requirements of women are greatly increased by pregnancy, maternity and lactation. Before birth and for months afterward the demand of the child is satisfied through the mother. Weakening of the bones and teeth of the mother, a common accompaniment of pregnancy and nursing, is due to withdrawal of calcium from these structures to meet the requirements of the little parasite within. As for "long-continued loss of calcium without the appearance of symptoms," I venture to say this refers to positive symptoms only.

Familiar positive symptoms of calcium deficiency include painful nocturnal cramps in the legs or feet, hyperesthetic rhinitis, machinegun sneezing, recurring hives, neuralgic headache, perennial hay fever and spasmodic asthma. Equally significant though negative symptoms are delicate, sensitive, unsteady "nerves," lack of will power, timidity, "weak backbone," and finally a proclivity to indulge small weaknesses, such as dosing yourself with aspirin, acetanilid or other analgesics for every little discomfort or using tranquilizers, alcohol or other dope to avoid recognition—and the need to face—shortcomings.

MINIMUM AND OPTIMUM   Nutrition authorities estimate that a sedentary adult requires at least eight grains, or about half a gram, of calcium daily to prevent positive manifestations of deficiency such as the symptoms mentioned in the preceding paragraph. This, remember, is the *minimum* for an adult who just sits and vegetates —at the office, school, theater, church, ballgame, in the bus or train, at the cocktail party, in the easy chair before the TV—and gets as little exercise as possible. A growing child, a pregnant or lactating woman, or anyone who is physically active, needs at least 12 grains.

If you worry along on the minimum daily ration—the amount you get from two glasses of milk daily, for instance—you accumulate little or no calcium reserve in bones and teeth. Hence if for any reason your diet is restricted for a while, as during the course of acute illness or a few weeks' confinement to bed, you quickly develop calcium deficiency manifested as weakness and the negative symptoms described above.

It is indeed my opinion that the peevishness and ill-humor of invalids unable to take a daily walk, or get any general exercise at all, is due mainly to calcium shortage.

THE FUNCTION OF CALCIUM   The functions of calcium in the healthy body are many. It is needed for clotting of the blood and for adequate contraction of the heart. It is essential for ossification of bone. It also diminishes permeability of body tissues and regulates excitability of nerve fibers and nerve centers.

Since we know that absorption and utilization of calcium is aided and promoted by vitamin D (see chapter on Vitamins) it follows that to maintain good calcium metabolism and good general health a daily ration of vitamin D is also essential. Very few of us get sufficient vitamin D through daily exposure to sun or skyshine. We must, therefore, take care to keep well provided with it.

Because it regulates excitability of nerve fibers and nerve centers, an optimum daily intake of Ca and D steadies the nerves and may be regarded as nature's own *tranquilizer*. Calcium and vitamin D used as a supplement to everyday diet (six Calcicaps or three Calciwafers daily) has brought so much relief to the pain of neuralgia, nervous headache, periodic sick headache (migraine), bursitis, lumbago, rheumatism and what the credulous call "arthritis" that I have come to regard it as nature's own analgesic. But mind you, all this is nutrition, not medicine.

Used as medicine, a single dose of calcium chloride or calcium gluconate or calcium lactate injected into a vein gives prompt relief to the pain of colic—gallstone colic, kidney stone colic, lead colic or the colic of black widow bite.

More commonly than most physicians realize the peevish, irritable, emotional state of the patient who has had prolonged illness is due to malnutrition, particularly long-continued calcium deficiency. This is at least partly the doctor's fault, for even if the patient cannot or will not follow a high calcium diet the doctor can and should insist on an adequate daily ration of calcium and vitamin D as a supplement. Aside from digestive disturbances which interfere with absorption and assimilation of calcium from food, and the low calcium diet *per se,* confinement to bed or chair aggravates the malnutrition.

Patients with hip fracture, for instance, begin to fail during the second, third and fourth weeks of immobilization. There is a remarkable loss of calcium—calcium excretion may be three or four times greater than normal at this time. An adequate daily calcium and vitamin D supplement would save a good many of these victims if some one would see that they got it.

Then there are millions of Americans, the 65 per centers as I call them, who are not confined to bed or chair but are virtually immobilized, say autoimmobilized, and hence, only a little less impoverished in calcium metabolism than the involuntary invalids. We'll have a hard look at these 65 per centers in another chapter.

The point I am trying to make here is this: No matter who or what you are, you can't get by without doing a reasonable amount of honest physical work. For a while you may kid your friends and yourself that you don't need any exercise, but if you persist in avoiding exercise, say by relaxing in the bar when you should be mowing the lawn, or riding to work or school when you should be walking, or sitting in the grandstand when you should be bowling or playing, you are training for a dull, short life.

THE HIGH CALCIUM DIET   The richest food sources of calcium —and we cannot repeat this too often—are milk, skim milk and buttermilk, cheese and green leafy vegetables. A high calcium diet is a health diet. For an adult it must include not less than three glasses of milk, skim milk or buttermilk daily. For a growing child or teenage youth not less than a quart, or four glasses daily.

Other good sources of calcium are peas, beans, cabbage, cauli-flower, broccoli, beet greens, turnip greens, collards, kale, okra, nuts, peanuts, oatmeal and plain wheat, egg yolk, olives and soy-bean flour. I omit spinach because the calcium in spinach is utilized to only a slight extent if at all.

Most Americans' diet of what I call "cheat-foods" is deficient in calcium as it is in other nutrients. Unfortunately cheat-food is cheap, plentiful in all the stores, comes ready-to-eat or easy-to-prepare and keeps indefinitely. "Just pop in the oven for a few minutes . . ." It is all too easy to eat and drink when you aren't hungry: candy, cake, pie, ice cream, sweet drinks may be gulped down without masticating—just what we need, since we are a nation always in a hurry. The sad results of such eating are demon-strated, for instance, in the large number of young men who are rejected as unfit for military service. While I am not implying that all this can be changed overnight by a high calcium diet or supple-mentary rations of calcium and vitamin D, I do believe that such corrective measures would be a step in the right direction.

The name of William Heberden, an English physician of the eighteenth century, is associated with little hard knobs, Heberden's nodes, at the sides of the end joints of the fingers of persons with chronic rheumatism—or rheumatoid arthritis, as some doctors call it. These nodes have also been blamed on "gout," that vague upper-class disease which to my mind it takes sheer imagination and nerve to diagnose. Heberden himself stated that his nodes had no con-nection with gout, which was a favorite diagnosis of his day, for they are found in persons who never had it.

Heberden believed, among other things, that angina pectoris was a cramp of the heart muscle. Dr. William Osler said a century later that this condition would be better explained as cramp of certain muscular territories, although he was vague about what these "territories" were. Today some physicians favor the theory that an angina seizure is *spasm of the coronary arterioles*. Others say it is due to transient ischemia, or failure of blood to reach the heart muscle. My personal theory is that if these spasms, cramps or contractions produce agonizing pain, calcium should be good for them and that a high calcium diet supplemented by an adequate daily ration of Ca and vitamin D would be good prevention. In an emergency an intravenous dose of calcium in addition to nitroglycerin or other vasodilator might be indicated.

CALCIUM CARBONATE FOR YANKEE STOMACH In horse and buggy days a lot of patients—well, anyway, some—would complain of hyperacidity, hunger pain, heartburn, acid eructations, waterbrash, uneasiness from fullness after eating, bloating and, their wives or husbands added, general crankiness. I mean they complained to the doctor: after all, why not when it only cost 50 cents and they expected him to throw in the medicine without extra charge. If the doctor tried to soak 'em 75 cents they felt robbed and next time would probably go across the street to the corner drugstore for a bottle of sarsaparilla. All these symptoms signify now exactly what they did many years ago—Yankee Stomach. I must add that in my lexicon any resident of North America is a Yankee.

Prescribing, or to put it plainly, handing out medicine, for Yankee Stomach used to be unsatisfactory and unprofitable. What with being routed out of bed nights to treat Mrs. Jones' son's croup or trying to find a "wood colored" house on a back road at night to attend a farmhand's wife seized with labor pains, I never gave much thought to the cause and prevention of Yankee Stomach until I took to writing and found myself with some leisure to meditate and study.

In the course of 20 years I eventually got back to a dictum of my father's—that all disease begins in the stomach. As a sophomore medical student I used to try to argue with him. "Not all disease. Take typhoid fever, where typhoid bacilli lodge in Peyer's patches in the intestine and . . ." Father would hold up a hand. "Then tell me," he'd counter patiently, "how the bacilli get into the intestine?" That to me was elementary. "Why, they are swallowed in food or drink." "And the infected or polluted stuff enters the stomach?"

Father drove home his point: If gastric juices were what they should be, they would destroy the bacilli and the patient would not come down with typhoid. Usually before I could think of an effective rejoinder the village jeweler, the county judge, the school principal or the minister would drop in for a game of checkers or a smoke.

In the course of twenty years I have reached the conclusion that Yankee stomach begins in the mouth. It is the penalty you pay for gulping too much unmasticated carbohydrate food.

For extraordinarily prompt relief of the *symptoms* of this, our national complaint, dissolve in the mouth or chew one or two Traco discs. Each such disc contains six grains of calcium carbonate and three grains of magnesium trisilicate, the most effective palliatives for hyperacidity. "Magic" is the word many sufferers use to describe the effects of Traco Discs on their hunger pains, heartburn, hyperacidity, acid indigestion or ulcer. But bear in mind the remedy is only palliative, not curative.

THE ROLE OF CALCIUM IN NUTRITION   When I was a medical student and later an interne our instructors used to say, "Study typhoid fever assiduously and you'll get a good medical training." This would be meaningless today, but at the turn of the century there was plenty of typhoid each autumn and our instructors were quite right.

Today, if I were a teacher, I'd tell my students, "Study the physiology and metabolism of calcium and you'll get a fundamental understanding of nutrition."

Now it should be common knowledge, yet isn't even among doctors, that if one absorbs enough calcium from day to day, it will do for the body what analgesics, sedatives and narcotics only *seem* to do. Sedatives and narcotics are half-measures. Calcium is the real thing. Unfortunately it isn't easy to teach nutrition to doctors. The science is too new, for one thing. For another, its newest knowledge comes largely from "outsiders"—neither Prof. Sherman nor Prof. McCollum, for instance, were M.D.'s—and for that reason the medical profession was at first inclined to pooh-pooh their theories, thus keeping itself in the dark. Some of the doctors even lend their prestige—did I say lend? They sell it!—to vendors of cheat-foods: all those foods deprived of vitamins and minerals by over-preparation or long storage. They get away with this because the general profession doesn't know enough about nutrition to recognize the evil inherent in these practices. Be that as it may, those of us who do know cannot emphasize the facts enough: You've got to have calcium for nerve, stamina, backbone, courage and heart—heart particularly.

Calcium is a tonic to heart muscle.

THE MYTH OF TOO MUCH CALCIUM J. Dorman Steele, Ph.D., was the author of *Human Physiology,* a textbook that was standard in grade schools in the nineteenth century. A critical examination of the book does not tell us whether J.D. got his ideas about mineral matter in the bones, absorption of matter through the skin, catching cold and "keeping the pores open," from doctors—or whether the doctors got their notions from him.

Anyway, Steele & Co. explained that the bones of elderly persons were more fragile than those of younger ones because mineral matter in the bones increased with age. The truth is, of course, that the bones of the elderly are weaker, more brittle, lighter and softer because the mineral matter, in this case calcium, has over the years been drawn out of them to meet the demands of muscles, nerves, glands and other soft tissues and, in the case of women during and after pregnancy, the demands of the developing fetus and nursling.

From time to time some eager beaver researcher or laboratory investigator warns the world via press bureau dispatch about the dangers of getting "too much" calcium which, he implies without proof, may then be "deposited" in kidneys, arteries, heart or joints. The disastrous effects are left to the reader's imagination. I have scouted and ridiculed this myth time after time and to date no medical or health authority has undertaken to take me up on it. Every time the yarn is reprinted, however, I hear from readers who, after having happily supplemented their diet with Ca and D for some time, have suddenly quit lest they get "calcium deposits." Some are just scared, some are mad—they threaten to sue me if anything goes wrong. If I reply at all, my answer is brief and to the point: Sue and be . . .

Calcium is only deposited, or more accurately, calcification of tissues only occurs, as a *consequence of degeneration* of the affected tissues. Nature attempts to repair worn out or broken down tissue with plaster of Paris, so to speak, when she can no longer replace worn out or dead cells with live young cells able to carry on the functions of tissue or organ. This is what is meant by calcification. There is no scientific evidence whatever that "deposit" of calcium, or calcification, occurs in otherwise healthy or normal tissues as a result of taking "too much" calcium. The truth is, as anyone with an elementary knowledge of pathology will tell you, that calcification is indeed an advanced stage of the degenerative process.

It is remarkable that the researchers and specialists who get their names in the papers never specify just how much "too much calcium" would be, although one college medical adviser did opine that students who were taking as much as four glasses of milk daily would wind up with hunks of calcium in their arteries, joints and kidneys. Health and nutrition authorities, however, agree that every adult requires not less than three glasses, or one and a half pints, and growing children and youths not less than four glasses, or a quart daily to meet the requirements of good nutrition.

I have presented the facts. It is up to you now to decide where the truth may lie, and then to begin acting accordingly.

Chapter Six

IODINE:
THE LAST OF THE SPECIFICS

Some clever Englishman once said it takes two weeks to cure a cold which, untreated, lasts a fortnight. For that matter one would be hard put to name a medicine that is a specific for any *chronic* disease or ailment. This applies to the shamefully over-touted wonder drugs as well as to old established pharmaceuticals.

We must concede, however, that there is still room for argument about the efficacy of medicines for *acute* diseases or ailments. Acute illnesses are mostly self-limited, so, when such an illness has run its course, you may argue that whatever medicines you used brought about recovery or else that recovery occurred in spite of the medicine.

A specific is a remedy that prevents or cures a disease, says Webster, as quinine is a specific against malaria. In the nineteenth century there was another specific—now almost forgotten—namely, mercury for syphilis. Syphilis brought more patients to the hospital when I was an intern than typhoid fever, pneumonia and all other infectious diseases combined. Syphilis in the second stage, that is. The neurological and psychiatric department was populated with long term inmates in the third stage. Yet it was a long time before anyone questioned the efficacy of mercury.

In retrospect I am at a loss to understand why or how the medical profession ever accepted or went along with the idea that it was a remedy for syphilis. This was something we were taught by our professors, and as good apprentices we thought they knew what they were talking about. It never dawned on me until two or three years after I had entered private practice that I had seen nothing to indicate that mercury was of any remedial value against syphilis. Thinking about this—I had plenty of time to think in the first years of practice—made me unhappy; so far as I was concerned mercury was the last of the specifics, and without specifics to comfort me what could I say in my reports to the Chief of Staff?

A favorite method of administering mercury for syphilis was by inunction, which simply means rubbing into the skin. The use of this method implied that mercury is absorbed through the skin. Of course it isn't unless the skin is punctured, scratched, blistered or broken. Any mercury that is absorbed when *Unguentum Hydrargyri* ("blue ointment") or other mercurial salve is applied to the unbroken skin is absorbed by being inhaled—the mercury volatilized by the warmth of the body. The amount thus absorbed is of course extremely variable and uncertain.

For instance, the patient who bathed soon after an inunction washed away most of the mercury and inhaled very little. On the other hand, a man who applied blue ointment pretty freely (to destroy pubic lice), then went to bed and pulled the covers over his head, as some persons will, inhaled enough to produce salivation and other manifestations of mercury poisoning next day.

Besides being an unclean and ineffective way of administering mercury, inunction was and is a waste of time and money. If the systemic effect of mercury is desirable, although I'm blessed if I can see why, it can be obtained and controlled by precise doses by mouth or intramuscular injections.

Sometimes I wonder why it never occurred to me, in those days when I was in a position to observe the results in so many cases of secondary syphilis, that it never was cured. I talk here about the secondary stage because we seldom saw syphilis in the primary stage, when the symptom is a single sore or chancre which develops from two to six weeks after infection, at the point of infection, and persists for several weeks before the secondary stage begins with a rash which, more often than not, does not appear on the face. It was with the onset of the rash that syphilis sufferers generally came to clinic. As I said before, very little could be done for them.

Then in 1910, when Ehrlich introduced his salvarsan, arsphenamine, arseno-benzol or "606", as it was variously called, I was immensely relieved. The first of the miracle or wonder drugs, the manufacturers and their subsidized experts told the world, would cure syphilis in one dose. Dioxydiamidoarsenobenzol, they assured us, would destroy every syphilis germ (*spirochaete, treponema pallidum*) in the body—achieve the dream *therapia sterilisans magna*.

When the tumult and the shouting were over, it became evident that two or three injections into the vein would be necessary. Within a year or two various authorities were advocating at least seven, some urged 14 and many concluded that the course of treatment should be 21 injections. After still another decade bismuth, antimony, gold and what have you came into preference for the treatment of syphilis, the dream of *therapia sterilisans magna* having ended as most dreams do.

In 20 months of internship in a 400-bed hospital in Buffalo I saw only one case of malaria and in eighteen years of private practice in western New York only one other case—both in men who had lived for years in the South. Malaria was a rare disease in Western New York in my time and according to health reports still is—genuine malaria, I mean, microscopically diagnosed, and not a "malarial condition" diagnosed by conjecture.

Our professor was delighted with the hospital case. He brought groups of students to the patient's bedside to see the malaria plasmodia in the blood under the microscope. For a week or so the patient, a vigorous young construction worker from Alabama, obligingly had a chill every alternate day, with fever and sweat to match.

The professor begged us to withhold quinine and give the patient instead capsules of some inert white powder, so that all of his students might have a chance to see the parasites in the red corpuscles. In the name of the advancement of science we complied with the request. But the patient did not cooperate. In not more than ten days his chill-fever-sweat routine ceased and his rapid recovery made the professor sick.

Not only that, but it made me a therapeutic skeptic at the very beginning of my professional career. Maybe it served me right for withholding quinine. Had we given quinine in the regular way the patient's prompt recovery would have saved the reputation of the last of the specifics, or I should say the last but one. I then practiced eighteen years without a substantial specific to lighten the burden of skepticism that rankled in my conscience. But I also had to support my wife and children and by bitter experience I had learned that people who laud you for telling the truth call another doctor when they are ill.

I was disillusioned and feeling mighty low by the time the science of nutrition was born. That, as I mention elsewhere, was in the second decade of the twentieth century, with the publications of Henry C. Sherman's *Chemistry of Food and Nutrition* and Elmer V. McCollum's *The Newer Knowledge of Nutrition*. These two classics and the voluminous literature that followed made nutrition a respectable science, whether the medical profession liked it or not. The new approach fully compensated for my loss of faith in pharmaceutical remedies. For instance, in the treatment of chronic joint disability—whether you prefer to call it arthritis or rheumatism—the so-called wonder drugs so lavishly prescribed by the merchants of medicine give no lasting benefit, but correction of the lifelong nutritional deficiencies which cause the disability usually gives not only lasting benefits, but often also cures.

For years I have been trying to teach chronic joint disability sufferers how to correct their nutritional deficiencies, but the poor souls are hard to convince because generally they know so much that isn't so. They also infer from the window dressing presented by the specialist or "clinic" racketeer they have consulted that he must be extremely successful. So they are willing to go along with him on a trial basis and to experiment with the latest miracle medicine. This of course costs a pretty penny—advertising space in the Journal of the AMA being what we all know it is.

THE SOLE SURVIVING ALTERATIVE   I never have understood clearly what an alterative is supposed to be. Webster isn't of much help—he says an alterative is a medicine that seems to cause some change in disordered functions, presumably a change for the better. From old medical tomes I gather that there were scads of alteratives in the materia medica of the nineteenth century. Most popular were sarsaparilla, sulphur, cod liver oil and iodine.

Sarsaparilla and sulphur are forgotten. Cod liver oil is prescribed today mainly as a source of vitamins A and D.

Iodine or iodin appears to be the sole surviving alterative. As an alterative it makes little difference whether it is in the form of potassium iodide, sodium iodide, ammonium iodide, elemental iodine, mild tincture of iodine, strong tincture of iodine, compound solution of iodine (*Lugol's solution*) or iodized salt. Whatever the form, it is the quantity of iodine that matters.

Potassium iodide, otherwise called iodide of potash or KI, was the standard alterative in the nineteenth century. But we thought of it as medicinal. Now we know it is nutritional and we also know that every man, woman or child must get a wee bit of iodine or iodide in one form or another every day to keep well or remain in better-than-average nutritional condition, which I call VITE. Iodine alone will not maintain or restore VITE, but as described in Chapter I it is one of the *7 Keys to VITE*. That bit of iodine which is essential for everybody is what I call The Iodine Ration.

Some physicians find it hard to regard this minimum daily iodine ration as a *nutritional requirement*. Being ignorant of nutrition they are pertinacious about it, for it is traditional for the medical profession arbitrarily to reject new ideas, methods, developments or principles. They feel their oats and so bray loudly that people get all the minerals and vitamins they need from a balanced diet of ordinary victuals—whatever that may mean.

Here I must make it quite clear, however, that no one should take medicinal doses of iodine or iodide except by direction and under observation of his or her physician. Everyone, on the other hand, should see to it that he gets an adequate daily ration of nutritional iodine.

The Great Lakes Basin and a strip of country across the southern part of Canada and the northern part of the United States is called the goiter belt because the soil, water and food of the area are deficient in iodine. So it is particularly advisable that people who live in this area supplement their everyday diet with iodine in one form or another.

Fish from the sea and shellfish—lobsters, crabs, shrimp, oysters, clams—are the best food sources of iodine. Preferably they should be fresh, but they are also good dried, smoked, frozen, canned, salted or marinated if the fresh food is not available. Vegetable or animal food produced on the land contains slightly more iodine in certain areas than in others, but never enough anywhere to meet people's nutritional requirements, especially those of school girls and middle-aged women.

Let me quote briefly from the reports of correspondents who take the iodine ration which I advise for everybody.

"We began taking Iodin Ration several months ago and now we hardly know ourselves. The improvement in my husband's disposition alone is well worth the price, and I have real eyebrows for the first time in forty years."

(H.H.R.)

"A few weeks after I started taking it I noticed how my hair glistened and hung so nicely, also was oily a few days after shampoo, whereas before it had been terribly dry."

(Mrs. P.J.)

"My daughter, 24, had always had straight stringy hair. Last summer her hair, on top, was taking on a natural wave and by Thanksgiving the sides as well were beginning to curl. Now it has a lovely wave of its own, without the aid of curlers . . ."

(Mrs. W.M.)

"Foolishly I let my Iodin Ration run out and within two months my hair became dry and dull, several white hairs appeared . . . now I'm back on Iodine Ration, hair has regained dark color and is shining again. I am most grateful . . ."

(J.S.F.)

"I had never seen gray hair get back its natural color, but mine did after using the Iodin Ration. I believe our soil (French West Africa) lacks iodin . . ."

(C.A.)

"Happy to report that since adopting the Iodine Ration as a daily supplement my hair has a shiny, healthy appearance where before it was drab and dry."

(Mrs. L.P.)

"Your Iodin Ration has been included in my daily diet for about a year and never before have I had such nice hair and so manageable. I am 58 and the gray hairs I had have disappeared."

(Mrs. B.A.)

"We live in the Great Lakes region and are users of the Iodine Ration. My hair was a startling white but now it's doing its darndest to be black again, its original color."

(J.W.)

"Taking the Iodin Ration two years. My hair, which used to be brown, has turned nearly black. Always had wavy hair but now it is curly, so curly that friends think I have a permanent."

(Mrs. K.R.)

"My hair has been restored to original color in the two years I have been on Iodin Ration. I can find no explanation for this except the Iodin Ration."

(Mrs. H.W.)

This is what people write me. For myself, please remember, all I can promise under any circumstances is that The Iodine Ration can do no harm.

Iodine deficiency immediately suggests goiter. A notorious lack of iodine in the soil and drinking water in extensive areas of the country (and hence also in vegetables, fruit, meat, eggs and milk produced there) is universally recognized as the cause of the simple goiter which used to be so common among school children before health authorities took steps to provide an increased intake of iodine for everybody, or at least for everybody who uses plain salt instead of iodized.

Not only simple goiter, or large neck, but exophthalmic or "toxic" goiter is due to iodine deficiency. Recognizing this, most surgeons make a routine practice of giving patients with exoph- thalmic goiter, or Grave's disease, minute quantities of iodine or iodides for weeks before and after operating. They have found that iodine improves the general condition of patients and enables them to stand the operation well.

So it is absurd to express fear or publish warnings against taking Iodin Ration or in any way insuring the intake of the quantity of iodine which nutritionists recommend as the minimum daily requirement to maintain good health. Some physicians and sur- geons obviously do not understand the difference between iodine in nutrition and iodine as medicine. One fine doctor feared there might be danger in using iodized salt and declared that anyway he didn't like the taste—but like so many others he failed to dis- tinguish iodized from plain salt when put to the test. He finally forgot all notions of "danger" after learning that there was more iodine in a single serving of salmon, fresh or canned, than he was likely to absorb in a month from exclusive use of iodized salt.

At our house we used iodized salt exclusively. Still, I doubt that I get enough iodine from that alone, so I take an additional optimal daily ration—an optimal ration being four or five times as much as the minimum requirement nutritionists estimate is needed to prevent iodine deficiency symptoms. In others words I take half a dozen Neoco-Iodin Ration tablets a day. Each Neoco Iodine Ration tablet contains one-tenth of a milligram of iodine, which is the minimum daily requirement. Should you already have mani- festations of iodine deficiency, I suggest one milligram daily for the first two or three months, or ten tablets a day. After that one a day may be enough to maintain iodine balance and good nu- trition.

Now for the dirty work. I hate to describe the general mani- festations of iodine deficiency other than goiter, but there is no way out of it at this point and so I shall carry on with the earnest hope that no one will find in it an excuse for drifting along without medical advice. I repeat that although one Iodin Ration tablet a day the year around can hardly do any child or adult any harm, if you find described here *several* symptoms that "fit your case," this by no means proves you should begin prescribing for yourself. Increased iodine intake may or may not be all you need to restore you to health and VITE. It is best to give yourself the benefit of a complete examination by your physician. Tell him in your own words what your complaints are; and only after he has told you what his examination shows and advise you what, if anything, you should do about it, submit to him the question of iodine deficiency and the possibility of taking on Iodin Ration.

Growing youngsters, especially girls in their early teens, who mope, feel too tired to work, play or study, seem pensive or even moody at a time of life when they should be cheerful and active, may derive great benefit from the Iodin Ration—or better still from Ray-D Tablets which supply not only iodine but also calcium, phosphorus, vitamin D and the essential B vitamins.

I know of one sixteen-year-old who had been under a doctor's care for a year for anemia. Treatment corrected the anemia, yet the girl continued to suffer from a kind of chronic fatigue which seemed impossible to overcome. This fatigue kept her from entering junior college. Finally her mother began giving her the Iodin Ration, and some time later reported as follows: "The result has been simply unbelievable. The doctor told me to keep right on with it. She is very happy and I am so grateful . . . she was so tired . . . great lassitude . . . she couldn't enjoy life as other young people do. Now she is bubbling over most of the time." Of course the family doctor ruled out the possibility of incipient tuberculosis before he instructed the mother to keep on with the Iodin Ration—any young person in similar circumstances deserves that break.

Just as many youngsters, more girls than boys, begin to mope in their teens for want of iodine, so do many mature adults have no pep or ambition, a tendency to doze off any time, anywhere, although they sleep long hours every night, put on more and more slack flesh, have a dry, sallow skin, lusterless, dry, falling, prema turely graying hair, and in some instances develop a melancholic outlook and manner which, to their friends, is completely different from their former cheerful disposition. These are common manifestations of iodine deficiency.

Anyone with iodine deficiency is likely to have a subnormal body temperature and to desire more clothing and greater indoor warmth than normal persons find comfortable. Their hands and feet feel cold, flabby and damp. They often complain that their knees are weak.

Adults in this fourth decade who have suffered from many years of iodine deficiency are kept from healthy physical activity by the persistent lassitude they feel. This inactivity favors accumulation of superfluous weight or bulk. Then, too, they may feel pretty good, warmed up and waked up, after a hearty meal; so they overeat. They also may get a similar effect from alcohol. But the more alcohol they consume the more calories are diverted into storage as slack flesh, pads of fat over collarbones and flanks. Then they complain that neither a good night's sleep nor a vacation seems to refresh them as it should.

Obstinate constipation and, in women, amenorrhea are also the rule. One woman of 40 reported: "A year ago I started taking Iodin Ration . . . vitally improved, bowels perfect, skin clearer and more life-like, amenorrhea of 14 months standing corrected, menstrual function regular for first time in nine years."

In children and adults alike, most of these manifestations of iodine deficiency occur without any sign of goiter or enlarged neck. Perhaps the occurrence of goiter in the school child or youth is an effort on nature's part to build up an iodine reserve, for the small amount of iodine in the body is stored almost entirely in the thyroid.

The unsuspecting drugstore customer who asks for iodine nowadays is too often confused and embarrassed by the reply: "Which kind? We have nine different . . ." Indeed, there are actually no less than five official, USP or BP or NF preparations of iodine in liquid form and at least as many proprietary solutions on the druggist's shelves.

But these are for medicinal purposes and should be used only under the direction of a physician. After years of vain endeavor to cope with these difficulties I have given up and now recommend only one form or kind of iodine for nutritional use—Neoco Iodin Ration, Improved. The name Neoco, identifies the commercial preparation I recommend, since in my judgment no other so well satisfies the body requirements.

It is the opinion of nutrition authorities that one Neoco Iodin Ration tablet a day should be enough to prevent goiter or other manifestations of iodine deficiency. I am no authority on anything, but I believe, along with Dr. D. T. Quigley, author of *The National Malnutrition* that "the quantities needed for optimum health have been very much underrated" and that where manifestations of iodine deficiency have already developed or existed a long time, a person needs from ten to one hundred times as much iodine daily as the normal individual who merely hopes to maintain fair health.

Chapter Seven

INSIDE AND OUT,
HAVE YOU HAD YOUR OIL TODAY?

In the New Brady Baby Book, I have this to say: "The first dose of physic you give the baby, under any circumstances, is the beginning of all the trouble you (and the baby) will have from then on. There isn't any laxative, physic, cathartic or "aid" you can inflict on your baby which is without a bad after-effect—binding."

By "aid" I mean enema (injection of soapy water or other liquid into the rectum) or suppository (insertion of an irritant, any foreign substance). Administration of any such medicine to a young infant upsets the natural physiological automatic regulation of digestion in the entire length of the digestive tract and makes establishment of the constipation habit almost inevitable. Indeed, I believe this is the way most victims of this bad habit get that way.

People of limited intelligence—and some who ought to know better—imagine that because castor oil is the blandest and least irritating purge we have, it is all right to dose oneself or others with it in any case of "acute indigestion." If the bellyache happens to be appendicitis, a dose of castor oil may convert a comparatively mild illness into a much more serious one, peritonitis, because more vigorous peristaltic commotion spreads infection from the appendix to other parts of the peritoneal cavity.

My memory may be hazy, but I think I remember taking castor

56

oil when I was a small boy. On the other hand I may only remember hearing my parents talk about it when I was older. Fortunately it did me no harm. The last dose I took—and I mean last—was some twenty years ago. The dosage was two ounces, which the doctor ordered for me the night before a G I series—X-ray pictures of the progress of an opaque meal through the gastro-intestinal tract. I was at the time being annoyed by frequent bellyaches that hampered my bowling. The X-rays revealed nothing but two or three dinky diverticula, or blind pouches, on the colon, such as many persons have and which aren't much trouble. Whether the bellyaches were from colic occurring when food or food residue happened to get into the pouches, I never learned. All I know is that presently they ceased and I have bowled and somersaulted happily ever since.

I do remember how pleased I was at being able to down that beaker of castor oil without tasting it. The trick is simple and I pass it on to you. First put half an inch of ice cold milk in a glass, then float the oil on it, then carefully add a little more milk. Finally take a swallow or two of ice cold milk, then quickly down the whole thing. Your money cheerfully refunded if you taste the castor oil.

But better still, try to avoid taking it internally altogether. Not that I am one hundred percent against it in any and all circumstances. Since learning to take it painlessly I am not nearly so set as I used to be against use of the stuff in therapeutics. Indeed, I recommend it as a remedy for the following:

1. *Warts.*   Once or twice a day apply a drop or two to a wart and gently rub it on (notice I do not say "in", for the fact is you can't do that). In two or three weeks, maybe, the wart will have disappeared. Of course, the way of warts is unpredictable —they are also said to disappear if you just steal a hunk of pork from your grandmother and bury it in the cemetery at midnight.

2. Sufferers from periodic sick headache, or migraine, and sufferers from neuralgic headache have found remarkable relief —for which I have no explanation—from a *daily* small dose of castor oil taken for many months, size of the dose to be deter-

mined by trial. Begin with a scant teaspoonful, always after breakfast. The idea is to take just enough to maintain as nearly normal bowel action as may be, but not enough to produce catharsis. Most persons reduce the scant teaspoonful by more than half in the course of the first week, then continue the minimum daily dose indefinitely. As already indicated, I don't know why any kind of laxative should help either migraine or neuralgic headache, but there it is. I can only say it is comparatively harmless to try.

3. Good emergency treatment for acute diarrhea from improper food, the trouble the old timers called "cholera morbus," is an immediate dose of castor oil to sweep out the offending or irritating food and then lock the bowel.

4. A few drops of castor oil may be added to a bottle of any alcoholic preparation for application to skin or scalp to prevent drying.

As you may have gathered by now, I have rather strong opinions about taking oil or for that matter any form of laxative or physic to keep the bowels "regular."

MINERAL OIL IS BAD MEDICINE   For one much given to name-calling, I confess I haven't even a suitable name for the poor gink who habitually takes mineral oil as an "internal lubricant."

It was the British Dr. Lane who, unwittingly no doubt, made millions of persons who might otherwise have enjoyed fair health become victims of malnutrition when he introduced the use of mineral oil (liquid petrolatum, paraffin oil, Russian oil, American oil, rock oil) in the treatment of constipation. The half-baked intelligentsia accepted without question the suggestion that mineral oil served a good purpose.

The truth is exactly the opposite. Mineral oil retards digestion by coating particles of food and interfering with absorption of the products of digestion. It also interferes with the absorption of minerals, especially calcium and phosphorus. It prevents reabsorption of bile from the intestine, thereby lessening both biliary and pancreatic secretion. It prevents utilization of both vitamin A and vitamin E. These are the reasons why the use of mineral oil as an "internal lubricant" causes malnutrition. In many instances the habit of taking it has led to serious impairment of health and even invalidism. Fortunately there is no convincing evidence that its habitual use contributes to the development of cancer, but I for one would be for abandoning it forever as a household standby.

Other oils, however, have their very valid uses both in the diet and in the home pharmacopoeia. Unfortunately some people don't distinguish clearly which purpose is which.

COD LIVER OIL ISN'T MEDICINE   Only two of the remedies widely used for chronic rheumatism in horse and buggy days are at all popular today. The two are cod liver oil and iodine. I shall discuss both again in my chapter on "Rheumatiz" but some of what I have to say about both is pertinent here. Iodine as a remedy for rheumatism was generally used in the form of KI—potassium iodide, iodide of potash—on the theory that it was an "alterative." It was thought then that alteratives produced a favorable change in disordered functions, that they corrected faulty metabolism. Sometimes, if the patient happened to suffer from iodine deficiency as most Americans did and still do, the treatment he got probably did him some good—provided he wasn't given too much iodine.

If I were suffering from chronic joint disability of insidious onset and long standing—in other words, rheumatism—and could only have one remedy, I'd plump for plain cod liver oil at the rate of one ounce, or two tablespoonfuls, daily the year around except for a few weeks during extremely warm weather. After all, European fishwives, or rather the wives of European fishermen, learned a long time ago that a snifter of cod liver oil a day kept their husbands from getting laid up with joint complaints. Now don't get any wrong notions: neither cod liver oil nor any other oil, whether taken internally or externally, "lubricates" the joints. There is nothing in the joints remotely like "oil," either in health or illness. If cod liver oil prevents rheumatism, it is because it happens to be a rich source of vitamin D and a good source of iodine. Deficiencies of both through the years permit rheumatism to develop—"rheumatiz" being *degeneration* of joint tissues. Cod liver oil is, in fact, the richest of all foods in vitamins A and D and also in iodine.

GOOD SUBSTITUTES FOR OLIVE OIL   Years ago when public health and medical authorities first advocated the use of iodized salt at table and in cooking, a colleague told me he didn't like the taste of iodized salt and neither did some of his patients. I may be singularly dull about this, but I doubt that anyone can tell by taste which of several samples of salt is iodized and which is not. A pound of iodized salt contains one part of potassium iodide in 10,000 parts of salt. A crony who is a chemist figured it out for me on his atomic weight computer: it would amount to something like one part of iodine in, if I remember correctly, 16,000 parts of salt. So I suspect my colleague and his patients read the label and imagined they could taste the KI in the salt.

The same goes for cooking and salad oils. I am happy with corn oil, cottonseed oil, peanut oil or sesame oil *in lieu* of olive oil. They are just as nutritious and digestible and a lot cheaper, and I for one can't tell by taste which is being served. By the same token, if butter is scarce I'll take oleomargarine. But oil I must have.

TO SOAP OR NOT TO SOAP   Whether to clean your skin with soap and water or with some kind of lubricant depends on the kind of skin you have. Basically what you put on it has a good deal less to do with your complexion than what you put in it. What goes into your skin depends on a number of factors—not only on what you eat and drink or are given as medicine but also on what you breathe, what sort of clothing you wear, how well ventilated your home is, how much exercise you get daily and how much sunshine or skyshine you give yourself the year around.

The coarsest, roughest skins, the poorest complexions, are generally those that get the least sunshine or skyshine. The skin of the patient receiving modern sunbath treatment for, say, tuberculosis of joint, bone or lymph node, as it gradually acquires a tan becomes beautifully soft and fine in texture and free from the blemishes that commonly appear on skins that are seldom exposed to sunshine. Quaint obsessions with imaginary harm done by exposure to sunlight keep too many misguided folk from enjoying the advantage of the cheapest and best of all cosmetics.

Some young persons have an old skin, thanks to bad hygiene. Some older persons have a young skin. A young skin has sufficient oil, secreted by the subaceous glands, to keep it soft, warm and pliant. An old skin lacks this natural skin oil and is dry, harsh, rough and irritable. A young skin may be vigorously washed with soap and water daily. An old skin should rather be cleansed with a bland oil such as olive oil, almond oil or sesame oil or with pure freshly made cold cream—cream made up by any pharmacist according to the standard formula for *Ointment of Rose Water (Unguentum Aquae Rosae)* given in the U.S. or the British Pharmacopoeia. It is a mistake for one with a young skin to begin using creams or oily or greasy cosmetics of any kind. It is unwise for one with an old skin to use soap and water, or in some circumstances even water alone, for cleansing the face.

Old skins give more trouble in winter, not because of the cold but because the indoor air in winter is usually excessively dried out by artificial heating and the skin suffers as do book bindings, growing plants, musical instruments and furniture. In the winter season an old skin needs a daily ration of oil to keep it in more supple condition. But air conditioning, or at least provision for the evaporation of several gallons of water in the heated air every day, is the best protection for old skins.

Contrary to popular belief, dust, grime, soil or dirt on the skin do little or no harm. Often the means used to remove them may be more injurious to the complexion. Nor do they cause blackheads or pimples. Plain soap, not medicated, is probably the best of all antiseptics or disinfectants to use.

SURCEASE FROM XEROSIS Noah Webster says, and this time I agree, that xerosis (pronounced zerosis) is abnormal dryness of the skin or eyes. Xeroderma (pronounced zeroderma) is a disease of the skin characterized by dryness and roughness and a fine scaly desquamation.

Xerosis and xeroderma refer to no specific skin disease but to a common state of the skin associated with various specific diseases and a still more frequent complaint of individuals who have no definite disease but merely some slight nutritional deficiency or departure from optimal health. Thus xerosis is the salient feature of ichthyosis (fish skin disease, alligator hide) and of psoriasis. It occurs in most cases of chronic eczema. It is also a normal evolutionary change in the skin as it ages. A young skin is soft, warm, moist or even slightly greasy, smooth, clear; an old skin is harsh, cold, dry, perhaps inclined to crack or scale, rough, dull, sallow or gray. A bit of skin oil or some other simple precaution to prevent excessive dryness can make a lot of difference.

Diagnosis and treatment of actual skin diseases is best left to the patient's own physician. The physician may not have a specific remedy or treatment for each disease, but mere failure to apply rational treatment or the ill-advised application of a wrong remedy may greatly aggravate or prolong the trouble. As in so many other instances, self-diagnosis may mean new problems.

The recipes or formulas suggested in this chapter are useful in a general way for alleviating xerosis or xeroderma and may be used indiscriminately. They are not, however, adequate treatment or remedies for skin diseases and should not be substituted for them.

Probably the most popular skin oil throughout the world is cold cream. Its official name, as I have already mentioned, is *Unguentum Aquae Rosae,* or in France *Cérat cosmétique* or *Crème froide.* It is most satisfactory when freshly made up by the pharmacist in reasonably quantity: keep a small jar on hand and the rest in the refrigerator.

For those who wish to mix their own cold cream, here is, approximately, the standard Pharmacopoeia recipe:

Pare into fine shavings one ounce of spermaceti and one ounce of white wax (beeswax bleached white) and melt them together over moderate heat. Then add 5 ounces of pressed oil of almond. Dissolve 20 grains of sodium borate (borax) in 1½ ounces of stronger rose water and add to the other mixture. Stir rapidly and continuously, or beat with egg beater or heavy spoon, until mixture becomes uniformly soft and creamy.

Cold cream thus freshly made, neither long stored nor made of petroleum products, serves every purpose a cream, cerate or oil can in the cleansing, protection or beautifying of the skin. It also relieves chapping, irritation, itching and sunburn. In other words, it helps to keep the skin young.

SMOOTH, SOFT, CLEAR SKIN   While the regular use of freshly made cold cream is standard for helping a dry, rough, irritable and lusterless skin, many victims of xerosis prefer the daily use of some simple neutral bland oil such as olive oil, almond oil, coconut oil, cacao oil (commonly known as cocoa butter and obtained from the cocoa bean, from which chocolate is made) and sesame oil.

Sesame oil, or *Oleum Sesami,* commonly called teel oil, benne oil or oil of til, is pressed from the seeds of the benne plant which grows in our southern states, in India and in other southern countries. It is as nutritious and digestible as olive oil and has two properties that give it preeminence in cosmetology: it keeps well without becoming rancid, and it does not clog the skin as do other oils. A few drops daily of the following preparation will be found an excellent conditioner:

SKIN OIL

> Heat moderately for three hours in a double boiler or water bath four ounces of sesame oil and 20 grains of powdered benzoin. Then let cool, add 20 drops of pure grain alcohol, stir well and finally filter or strain through silk.

Xerosis or xeroderma is known as ichthyosis (fish skin disease or alligator hide) when it becomes so pronounced as to have a scaly appearance. Backs of elbows, outer surfaces of knees and calves are the areas most commonly affected. The skin becomes dry, harsh, rough, scaly and in some instances shows a furfuraceous desquamation or peeling of the scales. It looks sallow and dirty. It is most troublesome in winter and in cold climates.

The daily application of skin oil and avoidance of soap and other irritants controls the trouble in mild cases. In more obstinate ones medical treatment is required. This means regulation of faulty functioning of the endocrine glands, and may include alkaline baths, sun baths and an optimal daily ration of the sunshine vitamin D.

Addition of 30 grains of salicylic acid to the *Skin Oil* recipe given above makes an even more effective application for obstinate patches of alligator hide about elbows or knees. Skin Oil without the salicylic acid is effective when applied sparingly to the scalp to correct excessive dryness after a shampoo. Simply part the hair here and there and rub a few drops of the oil on the scalp with the fingertips or spray forcibly from an atomizer with the tip in contact with the scalp.

Sesame oil has been used for centuries and is still being used as a beauty oil by the Persians and the Egyptians. Incidentally, the head of a beauty shop to whom I once gave the recipe reports that her pharmacist makes up the *Skin Oil* by using 30 drops of tincture of benzoin instead of the powdered benzoin and the alcohol and gets just as satisfactory results.

BE KIND TO YOUR SKIN   Many individuals who have a dry, irritable skin, especially during the winter season or while living in a northern climate, suffer a great deal from burning and itching after bathing, with the discomfort sometimes lasting for hours. A cream the formula for which was suggested by the distinguished New York dermatologist Dr. L. D. Bulkley has given relief to thousands of such sufferers. Here it is:

    1 ounce lanolin
    ½ ounce boroglyceride
    Enough cold cream to make four ounces of cream

If itching is intense, from two to four grains of menthol may be added to the formula: Label: *Skin cream, for irritation of skin after bath.*

For those who prefer a lotion rather than an unguent and for persons with a merely moderately itchy skin, the formula called "Dew of Sahara" is pleasing and effective:

    1 dram tragacanth shavings
    2 drams glycerin
    5 drops oil of bergamot
    1 ounce 5% solution (1 to 20 phenol solution) carbolic acid
    4 ounces sesame oil, or if not available olive oil
    Distilled or rain water, enough to fill pint bottle

Heat the tragacanth, glycerin and water together until a clear fluid is obtained. Cool, add other ingredients and agitate into an emulsion.

"Dew of Sahara" may be applied, a few drops here and there as needed, once or twice a day to any part of the skin by gently rubbing with the palm.

For chapping of the skin and to relieve redness and irritation from strong soaps or other cleansing agents or to stop the smarting and burning of the skin after shaving, the following lotion is generally satisfactory:

3 teaspoons boric acid powder
1½ teaspoons tragacanth shavings
1 tablespoon glycerin
1 pint distilled or rain water

Heat the tragacanth in the water until a clear mucilage is obtained. Then add the glycerin and boric acid. Label: *Skin Lotion*.

Apply a few drops of this lotion to the hands after washing before they are quite dry. Use twice or three times a day whenever the hands are red and irritated by soaps or alkalis. Apply a few drops to the face after shaving.

In all the skin irritations for which these remedies are used, irritations resulting from too much washing and bathing, from too strong soaps or other cleansers, the main cause is excessive removal of the natural sebum or skin oil. The cure, therefore, is to restore the oil balance. This holds true for men as well as for women—no need for a man to consider himself a "sissy" if he resorts to common-sense precautions.

No need for refusing to help nature along if your looks, morale and disposition are going to be helped as well.

Chapter Eight

INDIGESTION IS BAD NEWS

Once a newspaperman gets a wrong idea into his head it is pretty hard to knock it out. Years ago when the police picked up a man who was unable to tell them his name or where he lived, reporters informed the public that the man was suffering from aphasia. They even quoted the answers he gave to questions! I tried my best to tell them aphasia meant *loss of the power to use and understand speech;* that loss of memory, particularly of one's identity, was amnesia. But the word aphasia seemed to appeal to them and for years they continued to misuse it, oblivious to my plea that they check with N. Webster.

The same goes for the "acute indigestion" diagnosis. I thought for a long time that indigestion, like "catarrh" and "nervous prostration," had gone with the almanac . . . until President Eisenhower's first illness. I have always suspected it was the reporters, not the doctors, who labeled that indigestion.

Acute indigestion, if we are to be accurate about the term, implies that if anything retards or interrupts the process of digestion the patient is in serious trouble. Ordinary delay or arrest of digestion causes only slight discomfort and isn't in the least serious. I still remember how uneasy I was for the first hour or so when I was coming down with appendicitis. It happened one chilly autumn day when I had lunched on a hunk of coconut, then went out on my rounds. I gradually became aware of a increasing discomfort in my middle such as I had never experienced before. My stars, I thought, it just can't be that I, of all people, have indigestion! I was really worried.

I went straight home, crawled into bed shivering and waited for the doctor to come and make his diagnosis. Just being told that it wasn't "indigestion," plus the hypodermic the doctor gave me, made me quite comfortable, and the operation next morning and a week in hospital made a pleasant vacation.

Still, as I write this piece, I have before me a bottle of antacid tablets, Traco Discs, a combination of two alkalis, calcium carbonate and magnesium trisilicate. One or two Traco Discs chewed in the mouth (they are almost tasteless, and not at all disagreeable) will give extraordinary relief in cases of stomach acidity, sour stomach, heartburn, hunger pain, waterbrash, acid eructations, uneasiness from fullness after eating, bloating by gas or other discomforts from hyperacidity. So a great many persons have told me. Otherwise I wouldn't regard Traco Discs as superior to bicarbonate of soda or other antacids. All I know is what I read in letters from people who have found Traco Disks the answer.

In medical school my instructors used to allude to "dyspepsia" only incidentally, if at all. In current medical literature, textbooks and medical journals, only authors who are "way out" have much to say about the existence of dyspepsia. In the main, I learned about it only after I began practice, in Penn Yan, N.Y., population about 5000. There an aggressive charlatan was plying a brisk trade with the village dolts and the country bumpkins who came to town Saturdays to do their marketing and refresh themselves copiously at the numerous bars. The charlatan's ad in the village weekly newspaper identified him as, say, Joseph Sniggers, N. D., and I never did learn what the N meant. His customers thought they knew—to them he was Doctor Sniggers. Somehow they didn't interpret the sign on my office door in a similar way. They'd say, "Never mind about my diet, Mr. Brady. Just give me some medicine. Dr. Sniggers has already warned me about starches and fried foods."

J. Sniggers, N.D., was a tall, pear-shaped gentleman with several chins, flat feet and pince-nez complete with cord, and when he instructed you to avoid starches and fried food you were more impressed than you would have been by advice from any of the ordinary village doctors.

I was still innocent of dyspepsia and indigestion when I encountered my first detail man. A detail man is a traveling salesman who calls on physicians to acquaint them with his employer's product—mostly proprietary medicines which the doctor is persuaded to prescribe. The detail man's status has changed considerably in the past fifty years. Formerly he was primarily a sample distributor, peddler and order-taker. Today he is an instructor. You see, formerly doctors used to learn therapeutics first in medical school, then as interns, from demonstrations by physicians who had devised or developed new methods of treatment, and also by keeping up with current medical literature. Today the merchants of medicine just haven't time for all that jazz. Instead they make an appointment with the detail man who briefs them on all they need to know in one easy lesson. Then they prescribe his nostrums with little concern about the cost to the customer.

My first detail man introduced me to a certain new wonder remedy, supposed quickly to digest any starch that might cause trouble in the alimentary canal. I don't know just what kind of trouble it was supposed to be, but the detail man was as smooth as velvet—it seemed too sophomoric to ask him questions. Next day I gave a handful of the tablets to a patient whose symptoms puzzled me. She never came back, but her husband did about once a week for some more of those tablets . . . at fifty cents a throw, on credit, of course. I can't recall whether the bill was ever paid, but probably not. We remember pleasant things, but prefer to forget unpleasant details. Anyway, when I toted it all up I found that I had paid more for the new wonder tablets than I charged for professional services and medicine combined.

I did not sever relations with detail men until three or four years later, when one whose card said he was an M.D. came to me with a putty-like clay and glycerin preparation. It was to be applied, hot and thick, for various inflammations and infections. The "doctor" claimed it had proved remarkably efficacious for pneumonia and tuberculosis—when applied over the entire thorax and covered with a pneumonia jacket.

Pulmonary tuberculosis? I asked. Yes, indeed, incipient tuberculosis responded well. And the "doctor" went on to explain that the clay poultice on the chest induced a kind of osmosis which acted on the cavity. . . .

I had to interrupt the spiel right there. "You say you are a doctor, yet you hypothesize a cavity in incipient tuberculosis? That's ridiculous!"

When the detail man finally got it through his head that cavity formation occurs only in advanced cases of tuberculosis, he apologized, remarking that no one had noticed this before and the company would be grateful for my criticism of their sales argument. Whether the company revised the argument I never did find out. But I was amazed to learn just the other day that the goo is still on the market, a favorite medicament of Saireygamps and little tin doctors.

Since my unrewarding experiences with the new remedy and the poultice I have been as leery of detail men as I have of indigestion and dyspepsia. Let me pass my distrust on to you, even though it is against my principles to say anything that might frighten or worry anyone. If you find that one or more attacks or spells of what you think is merely "dyspepsia" or "indigestion" interfere with your work, play or sleep, for health's sake quit playing around and consult a physician.

I shudder to think of the prodigious quantities of stuff that have been swallowed by civilized American adults since the myth started that there is a magic substance called pepsin which will "digest" food whether the stomach is willing or not. It is possible that back in the Victorian era some eminent specialist (eminence being conferred on a doctor when he lends or sells use of his name to the promoter) really did imagine pepsin might do some good in some cases of stomach or digestive trouble. But in my own professional lifetime I have never known or heard of a reputable physician or specialist administering or prescribing pepsin as a remedy for anything. Moreover, normal secretion of pepsin in the stomach is rarely deficient as long as the individual can or does take any food at all.

Lack of pepsin, then, is seldom if ever a cause of "poor digestion," "stomach trouble," "dyspepsia" or "indigestion," and for that matter neither pepsin nor any other digestive ferment or enzyme or combination of enzymes would seem to have any remedial value in disturbances of the gastro-intestinal or digestive system.

An all too common cause of "stomach trouble" and "indigestion," a cause that is grievously ignored by most laymen and even by many physicians, is loss of one or more teeth and failure to replace the missing teeth with functionally efficient bridge, plate or other denture. This mere impairment of digestion in the mouth is bound to bring more or less disturbance of stomach and intestinal digestion, and physicians and dentists alike are derelict in their duty to patients when they fail to impress upon them the importance of maintaining good mastication and efficient mouth digestion. Digestion not only begins in the mouth but is conditioned by and dependent on the action of mastication and saliva on the food in the mouth and in the stomach.

SALIVARY DIGESTION CONTINUES IN THE STOMACH   This fundamental physiological fact is so often ignored both by laymen and physicians that it seems worth repetition. Good digestion begins in the mouth with mastication and insalivation of the food. It not only begins in the mouth but is conditioned by and dependent on the changes in the food which occur in mastication and in the action of the saliva, for these changes determine the character and quality of the gastric juice which will be secreted when the food reaches the stomach, as well as the length of time the food remains in the stomach before it passes on into the duodenum.

Without good mastication, that is, thorough chewing of those foods which need chewing, namely vegetables, cereals, cereal products, fruit and nuts, but not meat, salivary digestion can hardly be efficient. Salivary digestion is nearly if not quite as essential as stomach digestion. The digestive enzyme called ptyalin, secreted by the salivary glands, converts starch into maltose, a soluble sugar, but the action of ptyalin on starch is not limited to the short time the food is in the mouth. Ptyalin continues to digest or convert starch into maltose for half an hour to an hour longer before it is destroyed by the acids in the gastric juices.

Consider that about four-fifths of the calories in the daily diet come, or should come, from carbohydrates, in other words from the starchy foods, and that digestion of starch by ptyalin is as important as the subsequent digestion of starch and sugar in the intestine. Then perhaps you will acquire proper respect for and appreciation of the value of teeth or functionally efficient dentures. Good digestion, good nutrition, good health, V I T E, longevity and physical efficiency are simply unattainable without good masticating apparatus—your own or the dentist's.

ACID STOMACH IS NOT ACIDOSIS   Acidosis is a state of the body which occurs in the course of, or as a result of, various disease processes. I doubt that it is ever due to mere acid-forming foods, unless the diet is artificially or unnaturally restricted. Possibly the popular sport of tinkering with the diet may favor the development of acidosis in some instances, but we can't give much sympathy to people who attempt to doctor themselves when they are really ill. The common notion that certain foods make the stomach acid and also make the system, the body acid, is wrong. We can't go into the question further here, but I advise anyone with "indigestion" or a "bad stomach" to forget the acid producing food complex and follow a more sensible plan in the selection of food.

Nor is there any physiological basis for the notion, so much exploited by mail order fakers, that one must understand just how to choose the right "combinations" of foods—that's just sales hokum. Any combination of wholesome foods that suits your taste is a good, healthful combination to eat. While we are on the subject of food specialist quackery, let me say that all the "mineral food" rackets are for the gullible and the only nutritional superiority of whole wheat bread over white bread is the greater amount of vitamin B complex in whole wheat bread—which might be important if you were restricted to a diet of bread alone.

BANANA AND PLENTY OF IT FOR POOR DIGESTION   For years I have recommended (in the *Brady Better Baby Book*) feeding the baby banana daily from the age of four months. Especially the baby who has not thrived and perhaps suffers from chronic intestinal indigestion. This solves the constipation problem and makes the puny, sickly, malnourished infant grow strong and happy. This is the consensus or composite of a large number of grateful reports I have received from mothers who have tried it.

A distressing retardation of growth and development in infancy and early childhood is known as celiac disease, or as the venerable Dr. Webster insists on spelling it, coeliac disease. Celiac means a cavity, usually the abdominal cavity. Another name for celiac disease is chronic intestinal indigestion, and a common name for the retardation of growth and development due to the disease is marasmus, which means wasting, and the more familiar term for it is malnutrition.

In the American Journal of Diseases of Children, Dr. Sidney Haas published a report of his studies and experience in the treatment of celiac disease with banana diet. He concluded that the condition is due to inability to utilize carbohydrates and, to a certain degree, fats in the normal manner. But he found that carbohydrate in the form of ripe banana is "tolerated perfectly, making it possible to bring about a clinical cure in practically all cases. Whether there is a factor in the banana other than the carbohydrate which results in this cure is unknown . . . no carbohydrate except ripe bananas . . ."

Today we believe other factors in banana may contribute toward the cure of chronic intestinal indigestion and malnutrition, especially vitamin B and riboflavin. Banana contains also vitamin A and vitamin C.

Many adults subject to the functional derangement and nutritional impairment commonly mis-called "mucous colitis" have experienced great benefit from following a banana diet, or a diet in which banana is a large component.

Likewise the liberal use of ripe bananas in the daily diet has proved highly satisfactory in many cases of hyperchlorhydria or stomach acidity, even in cases in which peptic ulcer is known to be the cause of acidity.

Eat your banana and decide for yourself which of its virtues account for its excellent effects in chronic intestinal indigestion, celiac disease, malnutrition, so-called "mucous colitis" and acid dyspepsias. Among the virtues of banana as a health food these are significant:

1. Calories, 447 to the pound, compared with potato which yields 378 calories per pound.

2. Due to high proportion of easily assimilable sugars, the banana is excellent food for quickly available energy to relieve fatigue.
3. Bananas in diet tend to promote acidophilic type of bacteria in intestine, and to combat growth of putrefactive types there.
4. Bananas contain significant amounts of calcium, phosphorus, magnesium, sulphur, copper and iron.
5. Bananas have alkaline reaction and tend to prevent acidosis, and maintain a neutral or alkaline balance.
6. Bananas appear to increase utilization of lime from food sources of this element.

It is essential to select only well ripened bananas in any case. When a banana is ripe (ripening is prevented if bananas are kept in the refrigerator) the skin is golden yellow, flecked with brown spots (not black bruise marks). The pulp is soft, not mushy, yellow, not white, and delicious in flavor. The carbohydrate content of bananas in the green state, as picked and shipped, is almost entirely starch; this starch changes to sugar in the ripening process.

HYPERACIDITY AND PEPTIC ULCER So many sufferers from "acid stomach" with chronic or periodic "indigestion" learn eventually that they have peptic (that is, stomach, gastric) or duodenal ulcer and that special dietetic advice seems due these unlucky dyspeptics. Formerly, the Sippy diet was much followed, and with various modifications still is used by some physicians, at least in the early treatment. It consists of a mixture of equal parts of fresh milk and cream, three ounces being given every hour from 7 a.m. to 10 p.m. Between feedings the original Sippy method calls for large doses of alkalis—sodium bicarbonate, bismuth subcarbonate, magnesia—but this is not now regarded as essential, or at any rate the physician's own judgment should decide whether little or much alkali is advisable.

In a general way, the best guide as to what to eat and what not to eat is individual reaction. If you are unfortunate enough to suffer from hyperacidity, incipient ulcers or actual ulcers, you surely know what you digest easily and what gives you trouble. It is my theory that anything within reason is permissible in your diet so long as you are dentally equipped to masticate food properly. But whether an actual ulcer has been positively diagnosed or not, you will find that you get along better on five or six small meals a day rather than two or three large ones. This should include a snack in mid-evening and another just before going to bed; or you might prefer to omit the last snack if you have the habit of waking in the middle of the night with a slight sense of hunger or discomfort.

That familiar old home remedy, lime water, is sufficient to prevent or relieve discomfort or distress due to "sour stomach," hyperacidity, acid indigestion, heartburn, waterbrash, nausea in many instances, in child or adult. Anyway it is harmless. Prepare it when you need it, by putting a lump of live (unslaked) lime the size of a walnut in a quart or two of boiled water, stirring well, and letting it stand for a few hours in the earthen jar. Then pour off the clear liquid without disturbing the sediment. The clear liquid is lime water. Add a tablespoonful to each glass of milk or take it straight as an antacid. Lime water actually contains less lime, calcium, than an equal quantity of skim milk.

In general the victim of "acid dyspepsia" should give preference to fats such as butter, cream, olive oil, and to albumin or protein, such as eggs, milk, all kinds of meat.

Everyone whose diet is thus restricted should take regularly a suitable vitamin supplement because it is difficult to get the essential vitamins in foods such persons may take freely, such as B complex with iron and manganese in tablet or liquid form. If fresh fruit or fresh fruit juices or greens are not taken freely, some ascorbic acid (vitamin C) also should be taken daily, a tablet of 50 mg. Commercially canned tomato or tomato juice is a good source of vitamin C, when this may be included in the diet.

Many peptic ulcer sufferers can insure an adequate intake of vitamin B complex by eating three or four ounces of wheat germ daily. Even though eggs are usually allowed (egg yolk is the richest natural source of vitamin D), it is advisable in most instances to take some additional vitamin D supplement. Every physician abreast of progress is now prepared to advise and prescribe suitable vitamin concentrates to supplement a restricted diet.

EMOTION AND PEPTIC ULCER   There is still considerable difference of opinion among physicians in respect to the cause or causes of peptic ulcer, but most medical authorities now recognize that emotional or temperamental factors have a profound influence in many cases.

Characteristic history of sufferers is their relative freedom from pain and ability to eat anything when on a holiday; return of distress whenever they meet with an emotional conflict or mental strain or perhaps some business or domestic crisis.

Patients with peptic ulcer are generally of uniform psyche or disposition—highly irritable, sensitive, self-absorbed, mentally inelastic. Often they say they "swallow their anger," and in fact they are likely to feel a "lump in their stomach" when under emotional stress. Some physicians interpret these symptoms as pylorospasm or a tendency thereto, perhaps antedating clinical ulcer by several years.

Many authorities emphasize the role of tobacco in the causation of peptic ulcer. Especially in the young, and in the type of person who is by heredity or environment a candidate for hyperacidity and ulcer, autonomically unstable, excitable, energetic. The adverb *autonomically* refers to the subconscious, unconscious, involuntary part of the nervous system that controls body functions. Smoking on an empty stomach or before a meal is finished is especially harmful. In some cases the smoker suffers all of the characteristic symptoms of peptic ulcer, yet for a period of years, perhaps, X-ray fails to give positive evidence of ulcer. Tobacco is not only a common factor in the cause of ulcer but it is a major influence in preventing healing of peptic ulcer under treatment and in bringing a recurrence when the ulcer has healed under treatment.

Observation of a patient who had a gastric fistula (an opening into the stomach from the outside) by Drs. Wolf and Wolff showed that when a person has an emotional conflict involving anxiety, hostility or resentment, acidity in the stomach increases, motility increases, and engorgement or congestion of the stomach lining occurs, and these manifestations are associated with complaints of heartburn and abdominal pain.

Drs. Wolf and Wolff found that erosions and slight bleedings were readily induced in the stomach of their patient by trifling injuries (as by rough bits of food) when the patient was in a state of anxiety, hostility or resentment.

Good nature, good cheer, pleasant company at table make for good digestion and good health. Snarling, bickering, scolding, harping, complaining and discord at table spoil everybody's digestion.

ACID STOMACH AND GAS   During digestion and when hunger or desire for food has been merely stimulated, the gastric juice is acid. If this secretion of acid is deficient, the digestion of food in the stomach is retarded and the progress of the meal through it and into the intestine delayed. This subacidity or hypochlorhydria is usually present in anemia, chronic gastric catarrh or gastritis, in persons with vitamin deficiency and in some cases of cancer of the stomach.

If the gastric juice is too acid, on the other hand, the food is likely to be hurried through the intestinal tract before normal digestion is completed. Hyperacidity occurs not only in ulcer cases but also with gallstones, in persons who are excessive smokers and in some cases in those who are over-irritable or abnormally sensitive to everyday emotional stimuli.

Insufficient hydrochloric acid means that proteins are badly digested. Long retention of food in the stomach then leads to fermentation of sugars and starches and to formation of lactic acid and other acids as well as gases.

Heartburn, that painful sensation felt in the region of the esophagus, behind the breastbone, is due to regurgitation of even normal gastric juice into the esophagus or gullet; or to regurgitation of hyperacid stomach contents. It is pain caused by acid where acid should not be.

Waterbrash is the burning and irritation in the throat by normally acid or hyperacid fluid regurgitated from the stomach.

Eructation of gas, or belching, may occur with both hypoacid and hyperacid stomach. In some cases however the belching is mainly an unconscious, perhaps nervous habit of swallowing air and expelling it with sound effects. This is also the explanation for many "gas attacks" brought on by an emotional upset.

It is a common fallacy that such "gas attacks," or the mere presence of more than the normal amount of air in the alimentary tract, are dangerous. The gas is supposed to "press on the heart," interfere with, or threaten to stop the heart. No such thing ever happens. The worst that does happen is slight discomfort from the accompanying sense of bloat. If you do not let yourself become alarmed, the discomfort is presently relieved in the natural way.

CORRECTING ACID STOMACH   Stomach acidity may be caused by hyperchlorhydria (that is, excessive secretion of the normal acid of the gastric juice). Or it may result from fermentative acidity (that is, production of lactic and butyric acids in the undigested or partly digested starches and sugars which undergo fermentation when food remains too long in the stomach, as it does when the normal hydrochloric acid secretion is deficient).

The only way to determine the true cause is by a chemical test of the gastric juice or contents of the stomach an hour after a simple test meal.

If the acidity is hyperchlorhydria, whatever it may indicate, these rules should be obeyed by the sufferer:

1. Avoid all acids such as vinegar, pickles, sour foods.
2. Avoid all raw fruit except banana.
3. Take no soups or meat extractives such as gravies, consommé or bouillon.
4. For you all spices or condiments are bad medicine—this includes too much salt in or on food, pepper, mustard, hot sauces, catsup.
5. No sweets, no honey, no 'lasses, no candy, and reduce your sugar allowance to one-half the amount you have been taking —in or on any food or drink.
6. No alcohol in any form.
7. No tobacco.

Never eat hurriedly, but take time to chew your food well and do not wash down morsels with drink. In the healthy individual an important part of digestion of all carbohydrate food (sugars and starches) goes on in the mouth, the action of the enzyme ptyalin in the saliva. This continues after the food is swallowed. If the food is gulped down without mastication, the stomach and pancreas have an additional functional burden to carry. If the stomach is low in acid, the undigested starches and sugars undergo fermentation with the formation of gas.

If you suffer with even mild hyperacidity, it is a good idea to follow the ulcer regimen of five or six small meals daily instead of three large ones. But do not let yourself be intimidated into the belief that it follows you are doomed eventually to develop ulcers. Nothing of the sort need be true.

HOW'S YOUR GALL BLADDER?   Biliousness and bilious attacks were more popular a generation ago than they are today. The fact is most of them were caused by over-eating—the sin of gluttony. Hasty eating may, of course, have the same effect. There need be nothing organically wrong with you if you do feel this way—if you have been over-indulging. Nor is it a sign of danger to have a bitter taste in the mouth if you have vomited. Any normal person who vomits may bring up bile.

But if you suffer periodic attacks of "intestinal indigestion," as it is often called, with pain, flatulence or distension by gas and distress or oppression referred to the heart—perhaps even some irregularity of heart action—it is time to make sure you aren't suffering from chronic inflammation of the lining of the gall sac. Certainly if an attack is severe enough to demand medical attention, and especially if it is a repeat performance and you are "fair, fat and forty," gall bladder inflammation with or without gallstones is at least fairly probable. And if it isn't—well, allow yourself the luxury of ruling out any worry on that score.

Even though the gall bladder patient complains of "acidity," or "sour stomach," chemical analysis shows lower acidity than normal in about two cases out of three. The pain of inflammation is usually felt in the upper right quadrant of the belly or in the lower part of the right chest, and sometimes it is referred to the back under the shoulderblade. If you are subject to cholecystitis (gall bladder trouble) you should avoid all physics, for these will only produce or increase pain or colic. It is also common knowledge by now that you should avoid foods that consist largely of fat. In fact, all foods containing cholesterol, such as egg yolk, cream, butter, animal fats, vegetable oils, beans, peas, wheat, liver and brains should be excluded or kept at a minimum, since cholesterol enters into the formation of most gallstones.

I am convinced, however, that there is no reason to exclude from the diet of a gall bladder patient such foods as lean meats, cottage or Dutch cheese, milk, fruit and vegetables. I also recommend, as in cases of ulcers and acidity, the regimen of five or six small meals daily instead of several large ones.

RULES FOR RIGHT EATING   Whether or not you suffer from any of the difficulties I have listed, or are just interested in optimum health, here is a set of rules you may well find so useful you will make a habit of following them from now on:

1. Chew all carbohydrate food well. Meat or fat requires little chewing.
2. Always take a glass or two of water with your meals (this is contrary to the advice of a great many diet experts) but never use any beverage to wash down food.
3. Avoid extremely hot or extremely cold foods or drinks.
4. Never eat when emotionally disturbed, angry or worried.
5. Never discuss food, its preparation or its digestibility at table, and never permit others to do so.
6. The more of a ceremony you make of each meal, the better for digestion and health. At table good cheer must preside. Peeve, Grumpy and Co. should be strictly barred.
7. If your appetite is not good, rest a while before you eat. If your appetite is hearty, rest a while after you eat.

A sensible person is neither a vegetarian nor yet a complete carnivore, but a pantophagist, that is, he eats everything that is good to eat. It is foolish to avoid any kind of wholesome food because you imagine it is "binding" or "hard to digest" or "contains uric acid" or "is too fattening" or "is bad for the complexion." If one man's food is another's poison there's something wrong with the other man, not with the food. It is well to consider that most of the present beliefs and prejudices regarding food and diet are based on fallacious deductions made from casual observations. The dietetics accepted by the best physicians thirty years ago is obsolete in practice today, but much of this quaint lore is still cherished by the laity.

Whenever medicinal, X-ray, electrical, surgical or other treatment is advisable, it is conceded wise to leave the prescribing of the treatment to the judgment of the attending physician. That is quite as true of diet. If you contemplate any experiments in dietetics remember the fate of the tailor: Hearing how a big dish of pork and beans had cured the blacksmith of a dreadful gnawing in the stomach, the tailor tried it for his gastralgia and was already cold when they found him next morning.

And now, my friend, recall what I said at the beginning—digestion begins in the mouth.

Chapter Nine

STOP TIMING YOUR BOWELS!

Having traveled through Mexico, Guatemala, the Caribbeans, Brazil, South Africa, Egypt, France and England and the Mediterranean countries, and enquired carefully into the habits of their people, I can say with assurance that we Yankees are more obsessed with "regulation of the bowels" than anyone in the world. If you have even an elementary knowledge of the physiology of digestion, you will have to admit it is pretty stupid to try to "regulate" any part of the digestive process.

From the moment food enters the alimentary canal until the residue is expelled, the entire process is governed by the "sympathetic," autonomic, or involuntary nervous system, not by the will or consciousness of the individual. The only influence which the will or brain has is the initial act of swallowing and, later, the release of the "purse strings" or sphincter muscle which guards the outlet of the intestine. Even these are under voluntary control for only a limited time, since you cannot long resist the impulse to swallow food or water, nor long prevent the sphincter muscle from relaxing when the impulse to defecate comes.

Hence to think of regulating the action of the bowels is as childish as it would be to think it is necessary to "regulate" the action of the heart or the process of sweating. No sane person attempts to "regulate" heart action by means of daily medicine or other artificial aid. And any crank who made it a practice to take a mild diaphoretic daily to insure excretion of water and other substances through the skin in order to prevent injury to health because of retention of waste matter would only get laughed at for his pains. I hope you see the parallel.

My ideas and teachings in regard to this whole subject are based on knowledge and I assure you no scientific authority can or would controvert them. If you insist on disagreeing, that is because your ideas are based on misinformation peddled for several generations by quacks, nostrum mongers and ignorant laymen who have repeated it until even the charlatans themselves have come to believe it is so. Even some of my medical brethren who lack the time or the inclination to scrutinize some of these quaint and morbid notions have adopted them—but that too doesn't make them valid.

One theory that is particularly foolish is that of "autointoxication," which is supposed to be a kind of poisoning of the body by its own secretions. I wish to go on record right here and now and say unequivocally that, so far as our present scientific knowledge goes, there is no such thing as autointoxication or poisoning of the system from delayed or insufficient evacuation of the bowel. A person may experience some discomfort or even distress if the bowel movement is delayed for, let us say, a week. But that's the worst that can happen.

Some neurotics, badly educated by the pill and drug specialists, get into a dreadful state if there is a delay of even twenty-four hours in their bowel action. But the real cause of their malaise, headache and general wretchedness is anxiety, worry, fear of dire consequences. The quacks have got them scared silly—and scared sick.

WHEN THE BOWELS ARE BOUND UP   In his excellent little book, *Nervous Indigestion,* Dr. Walter C. Alvarez says, "Constipation is commonly of nervous origin," and goes on to explain how unpleasant emotions retard or stop digestive processes. For that matter all constipation is due to disturbed nerve-control. An example of this is the constipation which attends the painful condition called fissure or an irritable hemorrhoid.

People commonly speak of the bowel being "bound up." The great sympathetic, autonomic or involuntary nervous system controls the entire digestive process. The movements of the intestine are governed by branches of this automatic nervous system. One of these branches, when stimulated, causes contraction or increased "tone" in the intestinal muscle; the other causes relaxation or inhibition. The healthy, normal, happy, careless individual enjoying a good meal in pleasant surroundings, with cheerful company and no great sin on his conscience, giving nary a thought to the condition of his bowels, is never bound up no matter what he eats or omits eating. His internal organs function without interference for the same reason that his breathing and his heart beat keep fairly regular without any consideration or attention on his part.

Excluding, of course, such constipation as naturally occurs in innumerable illnesses where patients are restricted in diet and in other ways, we may safely say that 99 out of a 100 persons who are troubled with constipation are simply addicted to a bad habit. They need no treatment of any kind but only re-education and reassurance.

"So long as a patient is taking laxatives, hydrocarbon oil or bran," says Dr. Alvarez, "no one can tell how much his indigestion is due to disease and how much to the disturbing or irritating substances which he is pouring into his stomach." He declared that one of the first things necessary when patients complain of vague indigestion is to stop every form of treatment they have been taking for constipation. Alvarez takes plenty of time and space in his book to explain this and give illustrations. Since here we are unable to do the same, you will either have to accept my arbitrary assertions or shrug them off. You are the one whose health is concerned. But I must add this one suggestion: If such comparatively innocuous things as mineral oil and bran can produce disturbances such as Dr. Alvarez writes about, how much greater injury to health must there be from all the "vegetable" or "herb" physics which millions of misguided folk habitually take under the illusion that such crude irritants will "regulate" their bowels.

Mind you, I am not denying that poisoning from obstruction of the bowel can happen and does; but only if there is absolute or complete obstruction, not mere constipation. When intestinal obstruction does exist it is a very grave illness. Constipation, on the other hand, is merely a bad habit. If you happen to be plagued with it and wish to be rid of it, it would be rather futile to look to medication for help. The first step is to recognize that it is a habit.

Unfortunately for the health and comfort of the American people the dictum has gone out that a daily bowel movement is essential for everyone. To counter it, I suggest paraphrasing the old-time doctor's advice:

Keep your head cool and your bowels off your mind.

AUTOINTOXICATION IS AS RARE AS HYDROPHOBIA Of the occurrences of rabies (hydrophobia) in dogs and other animals there is no doubt, but I have never met a doctor who had seen an unquestionable case of human rabies or "hydrophobia." Even the classical cases reported in medical literature are open to a reasonable doubt as to the diagnosis. The diagnosis of rabies, in animals or man, is based upon the finding of more or less characteristic "Negri bodies" in the brain or spinal cord tissues, under microscopical examination. But these "Negri bodies" closely resemble red corpuscles in appearance, and therefore, the decision that the individual had rabies is a matter of expert opinion in the final analysis. I regard rabies in man as excessively rare.

I believe intestinal "autointoxication" or poisoning of the system, the blood, the body, by some vague waste substance or morbid matter or even germ-product which has been too long retained in the bowel, is actually as rare as hydrophobia or rabies. I am not expressing an idle conjecture or theory. I have studied this matter a great deal more carefully than most doctors have time to do. I have kept fairly close tabs on medical literature for many years. I have not found any scientific evidence that lends even a little color to the notion that you can be poisoned that way. On the other hand, I have observed much in actual practice that tends to show the absurdity of the theory of intestinal autointoxication.

THE DIET AND CONSTIPATION Back in the Victorian era doctors sometimes gave patients quaint diet lists, generally two parallel columns of foods, the first column items of which were marked "May Eat" and the other items marked "May Not Eat." Today nine-tenths of all the dietetic lore bandied about by various "experts" and gullible laymen is just as ridiculous as were the old time may-and-may-not lists.

Certainly diet has an influence on the function of the bowels. But I submit that as a rule of health or hygiene you should give no thought to any such influence. Even if this dish be loosening and that binding, what of it? Variety is stimulating in itself.

But I do insist that no food or dish or diet you can possibly choose is binding or constipating in effect. All foods or combinations of foods are laxative, without exception. Do not try to contradict me, because you cannot do it.

All that may be said with accuracy is, there is considerable difference in the laxative effects of various foods or diets. Some are more laxative than others, but all are more or less laxative. Just bear this in mind the next time you are prompted to avoid anything fit to eat on the grounds that it may prove "binding."

The least laxative diet is perhaps an exclusive cheese diet, though probably a diet of white of egg exclusively would be little more laxative. The reason why such a diet is not laxative is simply that it leaves so little residue after digestion. This is why an exclusive milk diet is not laxative. But an exclusive milk diet is certainly not binding, for thousands of babies thrive on it and hundreds of invalids subsist on such a diet without any trouble from constipation.

Do not tell me that such an exclusive milk diet is binding in YOUR case because it does not AGREE with you. You pay your dues for admittance here just like all the other folks and you cannot put on any exclusive airs over the rest of us. I am the one laying down the facts here, the physiological, undebatable facts, and your little whims or foibles do not concern us at all!

Of course any restriction, either in quantity or variety of foods in the menu, will produce relatively inactive bowel function. On the other hand, if a larger quantity or variety of foods be taken the bowel function will be correspondingly more active.

Those foods which contain a larger proportion of indigestible matter, such as fibre or cellulose, as in skins, seeds, coarse vegetables or fruits, leave a bulkier residue and that naturally acts as a more vigorous stimulant to the bowel. But I repeat, no one should choose or reject foods on that account, as a rule of health. If the victuals are appetizing, eat 'em and forget 'em.

As for "roughage," my own preference would be not to make any allusion to it in this discussion. But a few misguided souls here and there take such a morbid interest in it, as well as in the whole question of the "ease" or "difficulty" of digesting this or that food, that I don't see how I can avoid the subject. Let me say this, then: Anyone with ulcer of colon, intestine or stomach should follow whatever diet is prescribed by a physician. For everybody else my advice is, eat what you like whether it contains "roughage" or not.

Nor should the assumption, usually wrong anyway, that certain foods are "easy to digest" and others not, should ever influence your selection of food. By the same token I do not believe it matters in the least whether what you eat is baked, boiled, fried, roasted, stewed, well done, rare or raw—just so long as that is the way you like it. Enjoying your food generally adds to "digestibility."

ANXIETY PREVENTS DIGESTION In his classical volume, *Bodily Changes in Pain, Hunger, Fear and Rage,* Prof. Cannon tells of watching the stomach of a cat for more than an hour by means of X-rays. During that time not the slightest peristaltic movement appeared, because the animal under observation was worried by what was happening and probably a bit scared.

What is true of the cat or the rabbit or the guinea pig is true of all of us. Mere anxiety over the state of your bowels and about promptness is sufficient to produce constipation; so is anxiety or worry over any little or big thing.

Right here is the place for a little test, to determine whether you are likely to win your freedom from physic slavery. The most common factor of constipation is the habit of worrying over the action of the bowels. Your prospect of recovery depends on your appreciation of the pathological irony of that. If you fail to see the joke, just because you are the butt of it, it is too bad—you may as well go back to your pills, enema or gilded bird-seed and try to console your snobbish little soul with the notion that your case is different, your nerves, brain, etc., being rather weak.

The regular or periodic contraction waves that knead and mix the food and propel the mass through the digestive tract are called peristalsis. Dogs are not so "nervous" as cats, yet dogs in strange surroundings or in slightly uncomfortable situations show a cessation of peristalsis that lasts for two or three hours.

Similar effects have been observed in a few human subjects, though as yet science is handicapped through the lack of suitable human material for experimental study. Any kind of anxiety, worry, or fear, as well as anger, irritation, annoyance or other unpleasant emotion notoriously delays, stops or upsets digestion, takes away appetite and inhibits or retards peristalsis.

Even trifling anxiety, such as that about being on time at the office or catching your train or avoiding an encounter with your unpleasant creditor or keeping your wife ignorant of your gambling or your husband from discovering your extravagance, tends to slow down the whole alimentary function.

It is not as ridiculous as it may seem at first blush to say that a clear conscience and a happy disposition are the best of all aids to digestion and the only really satisfactory bowel regulators.

Of course, there are also prunes—but that is another story.

INSTEAD OF PHYSIC Whether you resolve to break the constipation habit or not, it can do you no harm to know that there are several good substitutes for physic, things which tend to favor natural or normal functioning of the bowels.

The feeding of a daily ration of ripe, sweet, raw banana to infants, especially puny infants with obstinate constipation, has proved a boon in thousands of harassed households, not only correcting the constipation habit but bringing a marked improvement in the infant's general nutrition.

Adults, too, should eat more bananas. A liberal use of sweet, ripe, yellow banana is particularly beneficial in cases of obstinate constipation of the spastic type or where there is a tendency toward mucous colitis.

Normal children, too, thrive on ripe bananas, despite ancient prejudices.

For every household it is good economy and good eating practice to keep on hand a pack of wheat. Its various benefits are discussed in the chapters on vitamins and on teeth, so let me merely point out that chewing it raw or cooking it up for cereal gives you the help of natural bran in digestion.

Many people are in the habit of paying high prices for a kind of imported bird seed, elegantly packaged and blessed by big-business humbug. You can get the same benefits from unground flaxseed which you buy by the pound from seed store or drug store. A teaspoonful or tablespoonful of it taken daily, washed down with water or mixed with jelly or breakfast cereal, provides a natural intestinal lubricant better than any mineral oil—if you need a lubricant. As a matter of fact the effect is very much the same as that of whole wheat, except that flaxseed is far less nutritious.

Finally, water is laxative. A glass of water on rising, before or at breakfast, after breakfast, and before, during or following every meal and the last thing at night, will aid digestion. Elderly or sensitive persons may prefer to take the water hot. The young and the vigorous will prefer cool or cold water.

GOOD NUTRITION AND GOOD DIGESTION   When the daily intake of vitamins falls below the level necessary for good nutrition, the digestive functions are all more or less weakened, particularly the motor functions of stomach and intestine. So that when trouble comes, rather than saying, "It must be something I ate," the diagnosis may well be, "It must be something I didn't eat." This holds particularly true when the trouble is chronic, develops gradually and is obstinate rather than severe.

In other words nutritional deficiencies, especially lack of vitamin B, are now recognized as a principal cause of weak digestion, poor tone in the muscle coat of stomach and intestine which permits dilation and stasis and, finally, constipation.

I advise every victim of the constipation or physic habit to begin, days or weeks in advance of the ultimate break with drugs, supplementing the everyday diet with an optimal daily ration of vitamin B complex in one form or another.

But do not make the mistake of merely "trying" vitamin B for a week or a month. Vitamin B is not medicine—it is essential food. If you take it at all, you should take it daily the year round just as you take protein or carbohydrate.

"One of the most constant results of eating food deficient in vitamins is colitis. It is so frequent that it may rank as a cardinal sign of vitaminic deficiency." So wrote Sir Robert McCarrison, world famous nutrition authority in his classic *Studies in Deficiency Disease*. He ascribed the "gastro-intestinal catarrh" which characterizes "mucous disease" in children to a diet composed largely of sterilized milk, artificial foods, white bread, polished rice, poor butter, overcooked vegetables and excessive quantities of re-fined white sugar in the form of candy, sweetened beverages and ice cream. For one thing such a diet is extremely poor in vitamin B. McCarrison attributed colitis in adults to the "long-continued use of deficient foods from childhood onwards."

In not a few cases, a half dozen or more somersaults on the floor or a mat or cushion every morning on rising, and some more rolls at night before retiring, have helped materially to re-establish proper functioning. This is no theory, but the practical observation of many years of experience.

HOW TO BREAK THE CONSTIPATION HABIT   Let us under-stand each other clearly. I assert that in 99 out of 100 cases, con-stipation is merely a bad habit. But I know that in the hundredth case it is due to some such real condition as fissure in ano, painful hemorrhoid, duodenal ulcer, or some abdominal or pelvic inflam-mation. In such cases, of course, nothing can remedy the constipa-tion but the cure of the pathological lesion which causes it.

We are dealing here exclusively with well folk who have the constipation habit. Even if the various medicines, freak foods, enemas and other articles habitually used by its victims were not in themselves harmful to health, it would unquestionably be better healthwise to break the constipation habit.

Now then, since it is mob psychology, so to speak, that gets people into the habit in the first place—along with an abysmal ignorance of physiology, as I explained earlier—it should follow that such elementary instruction in the physiology of digestion as I have just provided, along with a little counter-psychology, would break the habit.

If the victim happens to be you, do not let yourself imagine that what you are trying is a new and radical experiment. Thousands of others who were in precisely the same predicament at one time or another were able to abjure all physic, stick it out three, four, even five days—and win. It is all largely a question of intelligence and morale. If you are neither an ignoramus nor a gullible goop, you will not get panicky around the third or fourth day and will not go back to your old standby, the physic or the enema. Don't forget—that's what the quacks and nostrum-makers have been taking your money for all these past years—to keep you afraid of the bugaboo of "autointoxication." So exercise your brains, your character and your will: preserve a spirit of confident indifference and stop trying to interfere with a function that is autonomous anyway; and by the fifth day you will see nature resuming control, and forever after you will need only to leave nature and your bowels alone, ignoring the whole process except to answer the call of nature whenever it comes. And you will be freed for life.

This is the invariable experience of all victims who have the courage to stick it out, no matter whether the habit has existed ten or forty years, and regardless of diet, occupation or physical type.

Chapter Ten

BREATHING FOR HEALTH
AND LONGEVITY

A reasonable amount of general exercise each day builds or maintains health and prevents or corrects many common ailments. The reason is simply that exercise increases absorption of oxygen, therefore it improves metabolism. And metabolism is life —the internal combustion of fuel in cells and tissues to provide energy or power for all bodily functions including muscular work.

There is no exercise more beneficial than a brisk daily walk. Ideally the norm should be two miles of oxygen on the hoof three times a day, or else walking three miles each morning to office, store or school and three miles home each night.

By deliberately overbreathing for about two minutes it is possible to absorb more than the ordinary amount of oxygen. Try it and you will find you are then able to hold your breath for two minutes or longer, where normally a healthy person at sea level can hold his breath for only 40 to 45 seconds. Anyone unable to hold his breath for more than 30 seconds, I might add, is not a healthy person. If this is the case with you, you should consult a physician.

Yet from this it doesn't follow that it is possible to absorb extra oxygen hour by hour or day by day by means of constant deep breathing. It is actually impossible to overbreathe for longer than five minutes. If you try it, you will find yourself growing dizzy and faint. If, in fact, overbreathing for even a shorter period has such an effect on you, stop immediately, relax, perhaps even stop breathing for half a minute, then begin again slowly and shallowly. Presently the balance of oxygen and carbon dioxide in your blood will grow normal again—or whatever is normal for you.

Regulation of the depth and the rate of breathing is autonomic, or automatic, as is regulation of the volume or force and rate of the pulse or heart beat and regulation of the action of the bowels. If you have been led to believe you can regularly absorb more oxygen by breathing more deeply, or improve your circulation and make your heart do more work by taking digitalis, or maintain "regularity," as the euphemism goes, by the use of physics and enemas, you had better re-learn your physiology.

The purpose of learning natural, abdominal, or more properly belly breathing (from the Anglo-Saxon *belg, belig, bag, bellows*) is not, as some people think, to increase absorption of oxygen into the body but to free the circulation from the restrictions imposed on it by unnatural thoracic or chest breathing. Most of us have been taught from childhood to breathe the wrong way, through unnatural expansion of the chest. This badly restricts what physiologists call the *aspiratory* action of the thorax, or rib cage, since by rights the aspiratory or suction action connected with breathing should be the work of the diaphragm.

Think of the diaphragm—a muscle which works automatically yet is to a certain degree under control of the will—as a tarpaulin stretched across the torso between the upper and lower body cavities. Each time it contracts it reduces pressure in the chest cavity and increases it in the abdominal cavity. This lowered pressure in the chest enables air to enter—this is inspiration—and also encourages flow of blood to the heart from the great veins in the neck and arms, the abdomen and legs.

Each time the diaphragm contracts, it presses down upon the liver, gall bladder, stomach, spleen, intestine and the vast network of veins around them. But if you do not breathe naturally a large portion of the total volume of your blood stagnates during this process. Only if you breathe naturally, from the belly, does each breath pump some of the blood in your "middle" on toward the heart. Such proper ventilation tends to prevent many common complaints developed by chest breathers: varicose veins, bile stasis and hemorrhoids are the first that come to mind.

Primitive savages, children and a few civilized persons whose brains have not been addled by physical culture bunk breathe more efficiently and have greater endurance than ordinary folk. Singers, actors and elocutionists say that belly breathing improves their style. Persons who stutter or stammer report that belly breathing brings better control of speech and those past middle age find it tends to lower high blood pressure. "Nervous" people use belly breathing to get to sleep at night, asthma sufferers declare it keeps them more comfortable, young women with menstrual difficulties obtain permanent relief from it and victims of chronic catarrh in the nose and throat note a definite improvement after a few weeks of simple exercise that combines belly breathing and relaxation. The same is true for chronic liver and gall bladder sufferers and persons with chronic digestive disturbances. It also helps those given to much belching or hiccoughing.

Some authorities would have you think that there are two different types of breathing, both normal. One type they call costal, the other abdominal. They even may go so far as to maintain that the costal type is normal for women and the abdominal for men. This might have been true in the days when women's corsets gave them iron-bound waists and they had no choice but breathe through the chest or stifle—it is also the reason why they fainted at the drop of a hat in the Victorian era. But nowadays these artificial notions are no longer entertained by physiologists who know that women not hampered by freak dress breathe as men do.

Unfortunately most of us have been brought up to believe it is rather vulgar to have a belly and quite unrefined to let it expand even when we must breathe. And then there is what I call the chesty complex, the old sideshow barker notion that a bulging chest signifies great strength, virility, manliness and the like. Both silly myths combine to keep the front wall of the abdomen retracted or held in, and this false concept is preventing many people from enjoying the health that would have otherwise been rightfully theirs.

An exceptional case in point is that of the young engineering student who, along with a score of other youths, was being examined for physical fitness while applying for a coveted job. He stood out by reason of his fine physique and extraordinary chest expansion. Yet X-ray examination revealed incipient tuberculosis of the lungs.

It turned out that this poor gullible boy had taken unquestioningly and put into practice the suggestions of certain self-styled health experts that a large chest expansion "strengthened" the lungs. By diligent daily effort he learned how to expand the upper chest a good five inches as against the average two. He also absorbed other lessons, such as that ordinary physicians are all pretty dishonest and medical science is largely a lot of wild theories. He was so sure that fad foods, plenty of fresh air, cold baths and the exercises prescribed in the magazines would insure him perfect health that it seemed downright foolish to him to consult a mere medic when he developed what he called "a cold that hung on." Instead he wrote the health magazines for more detailed instructions about exercises, fasting, baths and so forth—and felt he was getting along famously when by sheer accident his disease was diagnosed.

But to get back to the physiology of breathing:

We have seen that the diaphragm, when not inhibited by faulty training, serves as a booster pump for circulation, aiding the return of blood through the veins to the heart, which then drives it on to the lungs for oxygenation. After inhalation has been completed, exhalation—letting out the breath or deflation—is purely passive, an elastic rebound without any conscious effort whatever. Drawing air into the chest—whether in the ordinary, automatic way or through forced, conscious, voluntary breathing—is the only active part of the process. Exhalation is comparable to allowing the air to escape from an inflated rubber bag. By muscular effort, principally contraction of the belly muscles, you can drive out some additional air after the normal quiet expiration has been completed. But this need not concern you here.

The Belly Breathing exercise which I recommend is one which many physicians prescribe for asthmatics and patients with high blood pressure. In both conditions the benefits are doubtless chiefly derived from the fact that the booster pump action of the diaphragm prevents blood from stagnating in the veins. From six to a dozen inflations of the belly each night and each morning should be extremely beneficial, not only for the various difficulties I mentioned earlier but also for such respiratory troubles as bronchial asthma, chronic bronchitis, emphysema or bronchiectasis.

Keep in mind that belly breathing is a study in RELAXATION, not an exercise in the ordinary sense of the word. In the beginning you should make it a practice to do all your breathing through the wide open mouth. In nearly all cases this is essential to promote the desired degree of general relaxation.

If I seem to harp on the idea of RELAXATION, it is because most of the evils of bad breathing are the result of a kind of muscle-bound state which chest expansion training has brought upon its victims. We know it takes may months of earnest practice to break up such wrong habits and free the diaphragm even partially from deeply ingrained inhibitions.

After several months of faithful practice it may well be that you will find it possible to breathe through the nose in the ordinary way. But this you can't decide until you have learned by long practice how to breathe naturally. Certainly no novice should attempt belly breathing exercises except with the mouth open, at least not during the first six months.

DIRECTIONS FOR BELLOWS BREATHING Try to forget you have a chest. Pretend it is paralyzed. Lie on your back, with knees flexed or legs extended, as you prefer. Let one hand rest on the belly to serve as an indicator.

Through both the open mouth and the nose draw in a slow breath, gradually inflating the bellows, as the steady rise of your hand will indicate, until you feel it is full. There must be no straining or extreme effort.

Now relax everything. Play dead. Allow the bellows to deflate automatically.

During this elastic rebound of belly wall, diaphragm and lungs, which drives the air out of the lungs automatically, you should be perfectly limp. When you feel that the bellows has been fully deflated and your hand has fallen as low as it will go without any straining or muscular effort, draw in another breath in the same way. Repeat from six to a dozen times.

Many persons find this bellows action so tranquilizing they drop off to sleep before they have finished a dozen inflations. For that reason it may be good practice to do the nightly stunt in bed. For the morning I would recommend the floor (with a rug or mat for protection) largely because body muscles relax more thoroughly on a completely flat hard surface.

If you faithfully practice belly breathing morning and night for a year you will surprise yourself by discovering how much more naturally and efficiently you breathe all day long. But constant consciousness of breathing is a bad thing for general health. Except during the exercise periods, I hope you are able to forget that you do breathe, and simply do it automatically.

BRONCHIAL ASTHMA Difficult breathing, short-windedness and wheezing commonly occur in cases of chronic bronchitis with emphysema (dilated or overdistended air-cells in the lungs), in cases of heart disease with heart muscle too weak to maintain circulation through the lungs and in some cases of chronic nephritis (Bright's disease) with uremia. Doctors have a word for this distress of breathing—dyspnoea, which means labored breathing. They speak of cardiac dyspnoea if it is due to impairment of the heart muscle power, or renal dyspnoea if it is due to kidney disease. This is not asthma, notwithstanding the careless use of such terms as "cardiac asthma" or "renal asthma" by old time physicians who were content with vague or confusing diagnoses.

True bronchial or spasmodic asthma is not due to any heart, kidney or other organic disease. It manifests itself in periodic seizures or attacks, like migraine or epilepsy, which last for hours or days, then subside, and examination of the patient's chest in the interval between attacks does not disclose any abnormality characteristic of the trouble. One may be subject to severe asthma yet in the interval present no signs or symptoms of disease to account for the trouble.

The important cause, if not the sole cause, of this mysterious malady is specific sensitivity to some protein substance which is absorbed through some other route than normal digestion and excites the typical reaction called asthma. Some persons have hives instead of asthma; some have both.

Every one has heard of persons suddenly developing asthma as a cat enters the room unnoticed, of infants who suffer an alarming digestive upheaval, asthmatic attack or outbreak of hives soon after receiving their first feeding of white of egg. Just why certain individuals are afflicted with such specific sensitivity we do not yet understand, but we do know we can test anyone for such sensitivity by applying to minute scratches on the skin homeopathic quantities of various proteins, then noting whether a hive-like reaction occurs at the spot where the substance is applied. Hundreds of foods, numerous animal hair or dander emanations, pollens, textile materials, dusts, fowl feathers, animal serums, germ toxins, insect venoms, plant extracts are employed in regular series for these tests, and as a rule the specific cause of the patient's trouble may be definitely determined by the physician, if the patient co-operates in the tedious tests. Once the specific cause is found it is usually possible to procure great relief and often a complete cure, either by removing the cause from the patient's environment or by immunizing the patient to the substance to which he is sensitive.

In some cases the source itself of the protein is a focus of infection, such as chronic sinusitis, chronic bronchitis with bronchiectasis (sacculation or cavity formation in some bronchial tube), or chronic tonsilitis.

Horse, dog, cat, parrot, canary, mouse, bedbug, parasites, geese feathers, silk clothing or house furnishings, camel's hair in upholstery coverings, glue, house dust are among the causes of asthma in some cases, as shown by skin tests. As already noted, the protein substance is absorbed through some route other than normal digestion; it may be through an ulcer or other lesion in the stomach or intestine.

RELIEF OF ALLERGY   In cases of allergy or peculiar hypersensitivity to such substances as dog hair, horse dander, pollen, goose feathers, dust, etc., the asthmatic attack may be greatly moderated or in some instances apparently averted altogether by prompt resort to Kalion Tablets (Neoco) containing potassium chloride and Vitamin C (ascorbic acid). Of course this remedy is in no way curative, but merely gives remarkable symptomatic relief. For this purpose the allergic sufferer may take two tablets *dis-*

solved—never otherwise—in a glassful of water whenever symptoms develop. This dose may be repeated three or four times a day if needed. Kalion tablets are usually sold in bottles of 100, but anyone subject to allergic troubles may carry half a dozen in purse or pocket for relief in emergencies.

It seems to be one function of some of the endocrine glands, particularly the thyroid and adrenal, to furnish to the blood a hormone or chemical agent which promotes the oxidation and destruction of foreign proteins or poisons in the blood. In some cases of asthma prolonged medication with the proper hormones gives great relief. In acute attacks a dose of adrenalin taken either by mouth or hypodermic injection, as a rule, helps immediately, though a repetition of the dose may be required at intervals until the attack is past.

Ephedrin, made from a Chinese herb, is now another popular remedy for asthma and its effects are similar to those of adrenalin. One of the most effective methods of administering both drugs is by applying a very diluted solution to throat and nose by means of a spray.

Ultraviolet light baths generally benefit the asthma sufferer. A combination of high doses of calcium and vitamin D is also recommended. Again, this means a diet of at least a quart of milk daily, along with all cheeses, egg yolk, carrots, cabbage, turnips, string beans, fresh, canned or dried beans and peas, oatmeal, oranges or orange juice, all kinds of nuts, all leafy vegetables taken preferably raw in salads, and finally plain wheat. In many cases additional calcium feeding is advisable. It goes without saying that along with the calcium some vitamin D should be taken to insure proper calcium metabolism. Di-calcium phosphate and calcium gluconate are the preferable calcium salts to be taken medicinally. These are combined with a good ration of vitamin D in the pleasant Calci-wafers (candy or mint wafers which children or adults like to eat) or Calcicaps (the same formula in capsule form)—such additional calcium feeding, regardless of the diet, should be continued for eight or ten weeks perhaps three times in the year—one Calciwafer (Nion) or two Calcicaps (Nion) three times a day.

These suggestions apply only to true spasmodic bronchial asthma. The treatment of other conditions attended with wheezing or labored breathing such as emphysema, bronchiectasis, some cases of heart disease and some cases of Bright's disease (nephritis) would depend of course, on what the individual patient's trouble might be.

It is my belief that weather, climate and altitude have little to do with asthma or its treatment. Generally the real explanation of any benefit experienced on change of climate is that the sufferer happens to have escaped exposure to his specific poison—say the horse, parrot or mohair sofa at home.

Finally, I think it is especially important that one subject to asthma should have an adequate iodine ration. Small daily doses of iodides have been used with more or less satisfaction as an "alterative" remedy for asthma for years. If you happen to be one of those persons subject to spasmodic bronchial asthma or to attacks of wheezing with intervals of freedom from the trouble, and are not taking iodine in any form, I recommend a very small amount to be added to your regimen—not as medicine but merely as an element essential to better metabolism and general health.

OXYGEN DEFICIENCY Total deprivation of oxygen or air results in asphyxia, which is apparent death or suspended animation or unconsciousness due to interference with oxygenation of the blood. Suffocation, drowning or inhalation of irrespirable gases such as pure nitrogen, carbon dioxide or carbon monoxide are common causes of asphyxia, which literally means absence of heart beat. Partial deficiency of oxygen in the blood or tissues is called anoxemia or anoxia.

Contrary to popular belief carbon monoxide gas is not itself poisonous. But it has greater affinity for the hemoglobin in the blood than has oxygen, and consequently when inhaled even in small amounts it crowds the oxygen out of the blood. The term carbon monoxide "poisoning" is a misnomer—the injury or damage suffered by cells and tissues is due to their being deprived of their quota of oxygen. Recovery may be complete once the proper balance is restored or the damage may be irreparable—depending on circumstances. So, poisonous or not, carbon monoxide is a threat.

Anoxia from chronic carbon monoxide gassing is far more frequent among city and suburban dwellers than most of us imagine. Its manifestations are often unrecognized or, more accurately, they are ascribed to other causes. How are you supposed to know, for instance, that the car idling in your neighbor's driveway directly in the path of the breeze blowing into your window is a source of lethal danger? It takes only one part of carbon monoxide in 500 parts of air to overcome the person who inhales it. Thus traffic cops at congested intersections, drivers in tunnels, persons entering large service garages, cooks and laundresses and tailors using gas burning apparatus and anyone carelessly using portable gas heaters may be exposing themselves to anoxia headache, at the least, or to faintness and being overcome, unless there is proper ventilation or air in constant motion around them.

Tightness across the forehead, flushing of the skin and slight headache are the mildest forms of anoxia. With heightened oxygen deficiency there is throbbing in the temples, weakness, dizziness, dimness of vision, nausea, vomiting and finally collapse. This is what sometimes happens to persons at very high altitude. "Pilot error" may be traced to oxygen deficiency at altitudes over 8000 feet and may well be the cause of otherwise inexplicable plane accidents. Now and again persons visiting at high altitudes make odd errors of judgment and a prompt return to near sea level may be necessary to keep them from experiencing what used to be called nervous breakdown.

Continued daily exposure to small but definite admixtures of the colorless, tasteless, odorless gas may give rise to all sorts of symptoms wrongly called neurasthenia, a rundown condition, overwork, fatigue and the like. Car sickness and loss of appetite are fairly common results. If you find you are suffering from a strange and unaccountable languor which is totally out of character for you, if you are pale but your hemoglobin is high on a blood count, you may be suffering from oxygen deficiency.

We know that monoxide anoxia is almost an occupational disease with iron and steel blast furnace workers, workers in coke or gas plants, workers in the garment industry, among linotypers because of type-metal heating kettles, among charcoal makers, miners, stokers, linemen working in conduits, porcelain enamelers and countless others. In many industries there are health law regulations that guard against it. But no such laws cover the tobacco smoker who deliberately saturates his blood with carbon monoxide. And no one bothers to tell the housewife who all winter has been working inside a poorly ventilated house, struggling with the heating system and spending hours over the kitchen range, that her "run down" condition by the time spring comes is due to a winter of chronic carbon monoxide anoxia.

If you have reason to suspect that you are a victim of oxygen deficiency there is a simple test you can use to determine if there is carbon monoxide in your blood: Dilute a drop of blood from ear lobe or finger tip with three drops of distilled water (which you can obtain by defrosting the refrigerator.) This produces a clear solution. Now mix with twelve drops of one per cent solution of tannic acid in water, and let stand. After a few hours it will show a precipitate. If the precipitate is brown the blood is normal. If it is pinkish-brown the blood contains carbon monoxide and it is time for you to do something about it.

SHORTNESS OF BREATH   Quickening of the breathing such as occurs with vigorous exercise in health or with slight effort or none in various diseases is medically termed tachypnea. It is to be distinguished from difficulty in breathing or labored breathing such as occurs during a paroxysm of asthma, which is called dyspnea. If the breathing is less difficult sitting up than lying down, as in certain cases of heart disease, laryngitis, aneurism and bronchitis, it is called orthopnea.

Perhaps the most common cause of shortness of breath, breathlessness on exertion or short-windedness, is simple flabbiness, poor nutritional state, lack of condition from lack of daily exercise. Next comes overweight or beginning obesity. Other causes are altitude, exposure to vitiated air (lack of sufficient ventilation in room), habitual or frequent exposure to air polluted with carbon monoxide, anemia, beginning diabetes and sometimes pleural effusion, which is an accumulation of "water" in one or both pleural cavities, with or without painful pleurisy. In a good many instances short-windedness is due to the habit of taking one or another coaltar derivative such as acetanilide in one of the numerous nostrums. In cases of acute carbon monoxide gassing, daily inhalations of carboxygen, three or four inhalations several times a day, will prove helpful. Practice of belly breathing three or four times a day is helpful. Where carboxygen is not available, breathing in a paper sack is helpful—the same method as that described for the relief of prolonged hiccough—hold an ordinary paper bag over nose and mouth and breathe in it for one to two minutes. This may be repeated three or four times daily—a practical way to get the benefit of carbon dioxide inhalations. Residence at sea level is better than residence at higher altitude.

In dyspnea from emphysema, (ballooning of air cells in the lungs) or from bronchiestasis (dilation of bronchial tubes) or in some cases of chronic bronchitis or asthma, the difficulty is chiefly expiratory, due to impairment of the elasticity of lungs and chest. The wearing of an elastic belt, band or corset around the lower chest and belly often gives considerable comfort and help in such cases. But even more beneficial is practicing the belly breathing exercise I have given you, since the trouble is not so much with inflation, which is fairly good, but with deflating the chest. That's where developing a flexible, efficient belly becomes an invaluable asset.

THE PROBLEMS OF THE SNORER   When we are asleep we breathe naturally, with the belly. A few adults do sleep soundlessly, but as a general rule the breathing of a healthy sleeper is audible. However there is a world of difference between the soft murmur of natural breathing and the distressing sound of a snore. The maddening part is that, like the skunk indifferent to its own scent, the snorer is not annoyed by his own snoring, though sometimes he does wake himself. Still, there is a moment at the borderland of sleep when the snorer may catch himself in the act if he has a mind to.

The basic cause of snoring is relaxation—the normal relaxation of the body in sleep, plus the relaxation, flabbiness and engorgement of mucous membranes of nasal passages and throat. This causes breathing through the mouth. The actual source of the snoring sound is the vibration of the soft palate flapping in the wind of the currents of air entering through both the nasal and the oral routes. Even worse sounds occur if the tongue drops back so that it obstructs the entrance to the windpipe.

When the tongue drops back and obstructs the breathing, the discomfort wakens the sleeper at least enough to bring his tongue forward again. If you are kept awake by someone snoring beside you, try to turn the sleeper on one side. If you yourself are the culprit, then keep in mind that the snorer who honestly wishes to overcome this can do a number of things.

First have a general physical examination. If at all overweight, set up a suitable regimen to lose weight. A reasonably daily program of exercise will help restore some measure of body tone and overcome the general flabbiness. In some cases a series of local treatments may prove necessary to relieve chronic congestion or thickening of the mucous membrane of the nasal passages; conservative surgical treatment for hypertrophy of turbinates may also be indicated. In some cases simple enlargement of tonsils and adenoids will call for sunbaths or optimal rations of vitamin D, or both.

If you snore, you should sleep preferably in an unheated room but always comfortably warm, and without heavy covers. Sleep always on one side, never on the back. Either use no pillow at all or the smallest pillow possible for reasonable comfort.

There is also the following routine of exercises you can follow, practicing at first in front of a mirror to make sure you are doing them correctly.

Contract muscles about the mouth as in a "prune" smile and "whew" and hold it for several seconds till the muscles feel tired.

Then contract muscles about the nostrils in exaggeration of the natural reaction to some unpleasant odor and hold it till the muscles feel tired.

Then the same with the muscles about the eyes as though straining to see something in dim light, and hold it for several seconds.

Then scowl hard for several seconds.

Then retract your ears or try to draw them up and back whether you can actually wiggle them or not. While holding them retracted, contract the throat muscles in the position of the "k" sound when you say "hike," and hold everything just so for several seconds.

Go through the routine regularly night and morning. It can do no harm, if no one catches you at it. But: Better lock the door when you do the exercises—if anyone surprises you in a seance you'll feel pretty silly.

NORMAL AND ABNORMAL MOUTH BREATHING Anyone running a race, fighting, climbing a mountain or swimming *should* breathe through the mouth. It is only while at rest that the breathing should be entirely through the nose. During any violent exertion a healthy person must breathe through the mouth in order to get enough oxygen to satisfy the greatly increased demand of the outer muscles, the skeletal muscles and the heart muscle. It would be impossible to get sufficient air by breathing through a normal nose under these circumstances.

Otherwise ordinary quiet breathing is better done through the nose than through the mouth because in passing through the nasal chambers the air is (a) warmed to more nearly body temperature or cooled if need be, (b) cleaned of dust particles which are caught in the normal mucous secretions of the nasal membrane, (c) conditioned as to humidity. If the air is too dry it is moistened along the way, if too damp some of the excess moisture is dried out of it. It reaches the lungs in the purest and best condition.

Habitual mouth breathers are more subject to throat, bronchial and lung troubles than normal breathers and this is attributable at least in part to the irritation produced by air that is not properly conditioned, as well as the more likely entrance of germ-laden dust particles.

Simple chronic rhinitis, hypertrophic rhinitis (thickening of the turbinates), polyps (usually secondary to sinus infection), adenoid hypertrophy and tonsil hypertrophy are common causes of mouth breathing. In children, however, it is well to take into consideration the frequently overlooked faulty development of upper jaw and teeth, which may require treatment by the orthodontist or any good dentist who straightens such irregularities of teeth, whether adenoids or enlarged tonsils are present or not.

It is a good plan to plug the nostrils with lamb's wool or oily cotton batting before going in swimming, or else wear a nose clip to keep nose closed, and breathe entirely through the mouth while in the water. This prevents many severe sinus infections in swimmers and divers.

A great deal more could be written about breathing, in sickness and health, but I have given you the outstanding facts you need to know. As you can see, unless there is something seriously wrong with you, a very little conscious effort will pay bonanza dividends in added well-being, a relaxed attitude and V I T E.

Chapter Eleven

EXERCISE: THE BRADY SYMPHONY

Metabolism, the oxidation or combustion process in which the energy stored in food or tissue material is converted into heat or muscular or organic work, is increased by exercise. The amount of oxygen your body absorbs from the air depends, as you now know, not on the depth of your breathing but on the amount of general exercise you take. The fallacy of the "deep breathing" exercises should be self-evident to anyone who has read through the chapter on breathing. You simply cannot hoodwink nature or amend the laws of physiology: if you want more oxygen in your system, if you want better metabolism, you must EARN it. Regular daily exercise is the easiest and best way to accomplish this.

I have already gone on record as an enthusiastic advocate of the daily walk. To estimate the equivalent of walking in terms of other forms of exercise is tricky, but here are some scientific observations that may help you evaluate your own activities:

Walking two miles an hour increases metabolism to three times the resting rate; walking four miles an hour increases metabolism to five times the resting rate. Dancing 15 or 20 minutes increases metabolism as follows: Waltz, fourfold; polka or mazurka, almost tenfold. The least strenuous dancing increases metabolism almost twice as much as gymnastic exercises; the polka or mazurka increases metabolism slightly more than running 160 steps a minute. I estimate that doing the "Brady Symphony" is equivalent to an ordinary two-mile walk in the effect on metabolism.

The Brady Symphony, by the way, is merely a group of exercises you may play anywhere, preferably naked, and always with the coldest air the season affords. It takes 15 minutes, more or less, to play the symphony through. Play it each night and morning, or at least once a day.

Before I go on to give you the exercises themselves, there are a few more general points I want to stress. First of these is the fact that possibly the best way to determine fitness is by checking your capacity to hold your breath. Holding the breath is a matter of the efficiency of internal respiration, that is, the capacity of the blood to carry oxygen, of the circulation to carry the blood, and of the body cells to utilize the oxygen and exchange their load of carbon dioxide for it. In other words breath-holding is an excellent gauge of metabolism.

Freak physical culture systems and methods involving exercises of great effort, such as weight lifting, overdevelop the skeletal muscles which, hypertrophied, become parasites in relation to the general body vitality, sapping it for their own nourishment. Such courses of training are ill advised, since they fail to develop constitutional vigor at the same time and also fail to train the heart and the circulation for coping with increased demands for oxygen and fuel. They only invite early physical breakdown and eventually premature senility and death.

Sound physical training, on the other hand, or to put it more accurately, sound physical education, develops constitutional stamina and promotes both physical efficiency and longevity.

PHYSICAL EDUCATION, ATHLETICS AND SPORT   Education is the act or process of training by a course of study or discipline. Physical education applies to the development of the body and the cultivation and preservation of health. The term athletics means activity or skill in exercises, games or contests. Sport is amusement, diversion or pastime especially as a spectator or "fan."

After all, for physical education value, no system of exercises, setting-up drill or calisthenics performed solo or in a group or class under an instructor or drill-master can compare with a game played against a single opponent or as a member of a team against an opposing team.

For years one fine high school required for graduation that the boy or girl candidate pass a rigid test in swimming and proficiency in rescue from drowning. That is what I call sound education. In another public school for years the principal staged private boxing matches or contests under proper supervision, and by such contests boys settled their differences or quarrels if any. The plan worked with great success until one spoiled brat boo-hooed to his foolish parents and they raised a scandal over the matter and succeeded in having the arrangement stopped. In my judgment no growing boy who has not received fair training and opportunity to practice the art of self-defense under qualified instructors who are members of the school faculty has had a fair deal in education.

Parents too often acquiesce or actively conspire with their children in various dodges to help the misguided youngsters evade part or all of the physical education the school curriculum provides. A favorite fraud is sometimes even aided by the doctor who in his abject anxiety to hold the family patronage consents to help a girl pretend a natural function is sickness, weakness or delicacy. This practice is a disgrace to intelligence. Doctors who participate in it should be exposed as shysters. Experience of thousands of young women of high school and college age has amply proved, beyond all Pinkhamesque eyebrow raising, that it is better for the health of the girl or woman that she continue all her usual activities, including regular exercise and athletics, without interruption during the menstrual period. There is plenty of evidence that pampering at that time, treating the function as a weakness or illness, invites trouble. Any boy or girl, youn man or young woman, who is able to be up and about should be required to take regular physical training as well as other classwork. It is high time that our physical educators put an end to this abuse.

BE A PARTICIPATOR, NOT A LOOKER-ON   No matter how loud you yell or how hard you root for your team, you will never become a hero sitting in the grandstand. Even a fraction of the time, effort, work and expense you put into such schoolgirl antics as becoming a cheer-leader would net you something far more real if put into playing tennis, baseball, softball, golf, lawn bowls, basketball—even croquet or horseshoes.

The vicarious excitement of being a spectator at the varsity game has been known to bring death to the old grad whose heart and arteries could no longer stand the strain. To be sure, sometimes a man dies suddenly while playing golf or lawn bowls or horseshoes. Still, there are more fatalities in the grandstand than on the playing field. And much of the "nervousness" of Americans is due to the prevalence of spectatoritis among people of sedentary habit. For honest working people, that is, for men and women who do get a reasonable amount of exercise daily, sport, especially open air sport, is a healthful diversion. For them an afternoon in the bleachers or grandstand helps maintain a well balanced metabolism. For white collar folk, executives, professional and other workers whose occupations involve little or no muscle work, sport as such is bad medicine. There should be a game for every such softie or "brain worker" with every player active in his game, whether it be figure skating, tap dancing or bowling on the village green.

Unfortunately for the peace and welfare of the U.S.A., very few general readers will comprehend what bowling on the green means, although the ancient game of bowls is still fairly popular in Canadian towns and villages, in a few northern communities and up and down the west coast of the United States.

Bowls is the game that held Sir Francis Drake from rushing to meet the invincible armada. It is played on a perfectly level close-cropped green or lawn 42 yards square,* with bowls built with a bias so that they roll in a curve. A set of four bowls usually cost less than $45 and last a lifetime or several lifetimes. A game may be played between single players, teams of two, triples or rinks, that is, four players on each side. Singles or doubles bowl with two bowls for each player; triples with three bowls for each player; rinks with two bowls for each player. Each bowler endeavors to gauge the speed and the curve or arc of his shot—the curve varies inversely with the speed—to stop the bowl at the precise point on the green where he wishes to place it. In tenpins or alley bowling perfect games are possible. In lawn bowling perfection is practically

---

* For details of construction of green and the game itself consult *The Modern Technique of Bowls* by H. P. Webber and Dr. J. W. Fisher.

inconceivable—and the unfailing fascination of the game lies not only in the lively, sociable competitive spirit it engenders but also in the constant endeavor to roll a perfect game, a perfect end, even a perfect shot.

And now to get back to our relatively unspectacular daily dozen, actually fourteen exercises or one better than a baker's dozen, which comprise the Brady Symphony. Even if you are reasonably tough it is a good plan to use a suitable mat or rug, at least two by six feet, for the horizontal movements. Wear as few clothes as possible—preferably do them naked, in fact. I have said earlier that I regard nakedness, not to be confused with nudism, as one of the seven keys to VITE and this is the time to explain exactly what I mean. A certain amount of nakedness is good for the body, for it gives all the cells a chance to breathe freely. Of course it would be even better if you could expose your whole body to direct sunshine or skyshine regularly every day, absorbing vitamin D through every pore and every cell. If, for instance, you had a flat, sheltered roof for exercising, that would be ideal. This, however, especially for city dwellers and those living in colder climates, is hardly practical. Just airing your body inside a sunny room will help.

If you are unaccustomed to active exercise, remember to go slowly at first. Do enough work to make yourself breathe hard, and puff and blow, grunt and groan, sing and shout all you wish while exercising. It is well to make your heart thump hard and fast for a while, well to get up a sweat. Open your mouth and breathe through it when you need more air. But always stop short of complete breathlessness or exhaustion and rest before resuming.

The natural type of breathing is of course best, so give your belly a chance! This is particularly important for young women, who are even less apt to breathe naturally than men. Fortunately young women nowadays manages to worry along without corsets, and the reform has proven a boon to the health and beauty of the sex. But there are still a great many girls who somehow have escaped physical education and most of these do not know how to breathe. They have not learned that the corset, girdle or brassiere which insures a woman the trimmest figure is the one she wears *under* her skin—the muscles of the belly and chest and back. A reasonable amount of daily exercise will keep these muscles in condition to give the most perfect support, at a fraction of the cost of harness.

TO SWEAT OR NOT TO SWEAT   Exercise that induces sweating is more healthful than exercise that does not, for sweating is a good index of increased metabolism. Sweat is practically nothing but salt and water, and contains too insignificant a quantity of any kind of waste or poisonous matter to consider. You may take a bath after the exercise period or not, as you prefer. The exercise period is in itself a cool air bath. I confess I am partial to dry cleaning; if you prefer a wet wash, all right, only don't let the bath cut in on your exercise schedule.

Illiterate persons generally undervalue the ability to read and write. Likewise persons without physical education—this class includes many school and college graduates, indeed many educators —are likely to deprecate and even disparage all physical training that claims a proper place in the curriculum. There is irony in this passive resistance to physical education, for the very word "curriculum" primarily means a race course, a place for running. He that reads ought to be able to run especially if he can't fight.

MAKE YOUR VOW, THEN PROVE YOUR WILL   Physical training develops character, personality, decisiveness, self-reliance. If your physical education has been neglected you may feel some such influence in yourself after a few weeks of even minimal daily exercise. It is easy at first to skip a seance on one pretext or another, but after a month of faithful daily practice, if you can manage to persevere so long, you will not want to miss a single play-time any more than you now wish to omit shaving daily, brushing your teeth, or dressing your hair. So, before you try the Brady Symphony or any other regular program of exercise, resolve as firmly as your flabby and undisciplined self will permit, to be faithful to daily practice for a month. I cannot tell you how much satisfaction you will derive from thus proving you are capable of self-discipline.

Remember, the Brady Symphony is merely a basic or minimal daily balance or compensation against the evil effects of "brain work" or sedentary habit; it represents the minimum daily exercise an adult must have in order to fend off flabbiness and unfitness;

it is scarcely sufficient to make or keep you fit unless supplemented by other forms of exercise, work or play.

You should realize that the hard breathing these or any healthful exercises produce is a natural and desirable reaction, for it means that the heart is being exercised and strengthened too. The hard breathing and rapid heart beat will both return to normal more promptly after you have acquired better stamina or "condition" through several weeks of training. Consciousness of this improvement is one of the rewards you will derive from this little course in self-betterment. Incidentally, let me assure you, a lot of gullible folk pay from $30 down to one dollar pinned to a coupon for mail-order "courses" that give the purchaser merely directions for some more or less advisable exercises and a powerful lot of general talk of doubtful value.

FIGURE OR NO FIGURE, DO STRIVE FOR GOOD FORM   Try to make every movement as accurately, gracefully and conscientiously as if you were participating in a public contest. Do not fool yourself by merely going through the motions. Strive for improvement in form all the time. But don't become too serious—there should be plenty of fun in the game for you! Many times when you feel brain-fagged, disinterested, dull, weary and utterly unable to do the evening's stint you will surprise yourself, if you manage to fight off the temptation to shirk, to find how quickly the exercises dispel the yellow streak and put you in chuckling good humor. I am sure you will agree once you have acquired the habit. The reason, by the way, isn't psychological—it's physiological: more oxygen, more pep, more life, more ambition, more contentment, greater joy of living.

My exercises are not intended for use in schools, business places or other institutions where large groups are involved. The exception is if the persons who exercise are given the opportunity to change clothes and, if they wish, to bathe before dressing again. When only a few minutes are available for exercise, I believe it is much better for a group of students, clerks or other employees to go out and take a brisk walk. It seems to me an unwise practice to attempt to put a class of school children through exercises in classroom or gym if they must wear their ordinary clothing. It isn't a fair deal either to the victims or to physical education. Movements 1 to 4 inclusive are suitable for schoolroom or office calisthenics, however.

SHOUTS, WHISTLES, WHEEZES, GRUNTS PERMITTED

1. BODY RAISING ON ARMS.—Place hands on floor fifteen inches apart, and hold body rigid on incline from shoulders to feet. Lower body till chest touches floor, then push up to starting position. Do once only at each session the first week, then increase one time weekly till you can do it six times if a woman, 20 times if a man. Breathe OUT as you lower body, IN as you raise it. (This exercise develops vigorous posture.)

2. SETTING-UP.—Stand erect, hands straight above head, palms forward. Breathe OUT and bend far forward, without bending knees, until you touch the floor with fingers. Breathe IN as you rise, with arms straight forward. Then swing arms vigorously outward and turn palms up, assuming semaphore position. Then vigorously resume starting position. Repeat three times at first, increase gradually until you can do it 20 times without fatigue. (For lithesomeness.)

3. SQUATTING.—Stand erect, hands on hips, thumbs forward. Breathe OUT and squat very low, so that your buttocks touch your heels and your thighs touch your abdomen and knees touch your shoulders, or at least strive for this. Immediately breathe IN and resume starting position. Repeat three times at first, gradually increase week by week until you can do it ten times if a woman, 20 times if a man.

4. SIDE FLEXION.—Stand erect, hands straight above head, palms forward, 15 inches apart, feet parallel, 15 inches apart. Breathing out, flex body sidewise at the waist and sway arms as far as possible to right, taking pains to keep hands the same distance apart at all times. Swing up to starting position. Repeat the movement to the left. Breathe out as you swing sideways, in as you swing back to starting position. Keep the head moderately flexed on the neck, not bent backward. All flexion should be in the sidewise plane, not forward or backward. Repeat this once the first

week, and once more each week until you do it 20 times without fatigue. (This is one of the hardest movements in the series, because it calls for use of muscles which you seldom use. It is of great value in preventing and removing pads or masses of fat from the flanks, sides and back, besides making the body more limber and supple.)

TO MAKE SHORT PERSONS SEEM TALLER   5. BACKWARD KICK AND SWIM.—Extend arms palm down and kick the right leg backward as high as you can, rising just as little off your heel as you kick and leaning forward. Breathe OUT as you kick backward with your right leg and throw out your arms as far forward as you can, palms down, in swimming position. Then breathe IN as you swing arms far out and backward as in breast stroke swimming, and draw the leg down to starting position. Repeat with left leg. Do once with each leg the first week, then increase each week until you can do each movement five times if a woman, ten times if a man. This exercise melts fat and develops muscles of hips and buttocks.

6. TALL STRETCH AND POSTURE.—Stand erect, feet parallel and 15 inches apart, chin in, chest up. Raise arms high above head, clench fists hard, stiffen your whole body except the belly, and breathe slowly IN. Make believe you are chinning yourself— pull the rigid arms slowly down, fists approaching points of shoulders, and then begin to rise slowly as high as you can on your toes, toeing in, and continue on down with the arms till you have in imagination pushed yourself up on a bar to level of your thighs. Slowly resume starting position as you breathe OUT. Repeat from three to 20 times. This is a hard exercise and, if done with the right spirit, a very valuable one for improving posture and carriage.

VERY BAD FOR THE CORSET TRADE   7. LIMBERING WAIST.—Stand as for No. 4. Swing body far over and down to right, bending as much as you wish at hips and knees and twisting body as much as necessary, breathing OUT, and strive to touch the floor behind your heels with your fingers, right hand behind left heel, left behind right heel. Then breathe IN, swing straight up again and down to repeat the movement on the opposite side. Repeat from five to 20 times.

8. COMPRESSION.—Squat, heels together, toes apart, head bent downward till forehead nearly or quite touches heels and crown touches floor, while you grasp your feet behind heels with your hands, your arms being inside your widely separated knees and your hands outside your ankles. Try to hold this position while you count ten.

The foregoing exercises, when you have practiced regularly for six months or more, are usually completed in approximately seven minutes, though they will require more time at first. They leave you puffing and perspiring a little if it is not extremely cold. The next six exercises usually consume the balance of a 15 minute period.

WE GO TO THE MAT   9. Lie prone on the floor, face turned to one side, hands beside head, palms down. Breathe OUT and give a kick or flop which lifts feet, knees and hips free of floor for a moment, the body falling to floor again with a slight bump. Repeat up to ten times as you gain endurance.

10. Lie in same position, hands on hips, thumbs forward. Breathe IN and raise upper part of the body as high as you can from floor without lifting feet, at the same time twisting your head about so that you see both heels and calves. Repeat up to ten times. Backs are strengthened by this exercise.

11. Lie supine, hands on floor. Without lifting head or shoulders from floor slowly raise both legs up to vertical, breathing IN; then slowly lower them to floor again, breathing OUT. Repeat up to 20 times, but only twice at first.

SIT TIGHT, THIS IS THE GRAND FINALE   12. Lie in the same position, hands on hips, thumbs back. Without lifting heels from floor, slowly raise body to sitting posture as you breathe OUT, and slowly back again as you breathe IN. Repeat twice at first and gradually one more time each week till you can do it 20 times without fatigue or cramp. Nos. 11 and 12 are famous for girth control.

13. FOR LOIN, GROIN and PELVIS MUSCLES.—This movement is the same as No. 11 except that the legs are carried over, hips and knees flexed, so that the thighs are momentarily pressed down upon the abdomen, then straightened up again to vertical and back to starting position—from three to seven times for a woman, from eight to 20 times for a man. This and No. 14 are valuable for anyone with slight hernia or tendency thereto.

14. FOR ABDOMINAL AND BACK MUSCLES.—This is the same as No. 12, except that the body is carried on forward so that the abdomen momentarily compresses the thighs. Return to sitting posture and back to starting position. Do up to ten times for a woman, 20 for a man. If hernia exists support the point of protrusion with your hand while doing exercise.

For people still fit or young enough to roll somersaults there is an additional exercise especially beneficial for counteracting the ptosis, drooping, sagging effect of habitual prolonged sitting or standing. Lie on the floor, bracing with outstretched arms, and raise your body as high as you can on shoulders and back of neck, then ride an imaginary bicycle for a while, say for ten to 20 revolutions of the pedals at each session, morning and evening.

If you feel ambitious you might begin the Symphony with half a dozen somersaults forward and, unless you are too old and dignified, backward, just to get your spirit moving. Finish the Symphony with some more rolls, of which more in the next chapter.

Chapter Twelve

THE BRADY SOMERSAULT

Somewhere along in the book I make reference to my father's delightful periodic lunacies. Everyone, I claim, is entitled to a few, my own pet insanity being somersaults. It may be that I'd be just as hale and hearty without doing them regularly, and no doubt many of my readers, and perhaps my own family, are sometimes tempted to chant, ". . . And yet you persistently stand on your head; do you think at your age it is right?" To which I would unhesitatingly answer, "You bet!"

Any eight-year-old boy can show you how to roll a somersault and come up on your feet smiling. If he can't, his guardian needs psychiatric advice. When I was a boy on Chapel Street in Canandaigua, every one of us rolled somersaults as a matter of course and some of us turned air-springs on Main Street lawns on our way to and from school. At least we called 'em air-springs. Noah Webster insists they are somersaults, but if you go along with that you have no choice but to call somersaults merely forward rolls—which makes the whole business seem as phony and confusing as a cocktail party.

If it has been many years since you indulged in any such monkeyshines, then it is the part of discretion for you to go at it systematically. In any case I wish to make this perfectly clear: I do not *advise* anyone to somersault, I merely describe the benefits I believe I have derived from forty years' worth of rolls before breakfast. If you still decide to try rolling your own, you will be doing

117

so at your own peril. And if I were you, and tried somersaulting on my own and came up with a wrenched neck or dislocated *derrière* instead of a smile, I wouldn't sue for damages unless I could prove the so-and-so *made* me do them!

I am reminded of the little student nurse who used to write in to say she found the information and advice in my syndicated column uniformly sound and helpful. One day I recommended somersaults for sallow complexion, cold feet, the blues and what not, and the nurse telephoned her druggist to inquire whether he carried them. He said she'd have to have a prescription. Another druggist said he had something better, a patent brand of effervescent salts. So the young lady wrote and asked if I would be good enough to send her a trial sample. I hope she was pleased with what I did send: Pamphlet No. 32, titled *Somersaults*.

To prepare yourself for your first roll, practice crouching and making yourself into the tightest possible ball, as though to fit into a hoop. In this position—on your toes, hands and the crown (not the top) of your head—it takes only a slight push of your feet to roll you over. Probably you will land in a clumsy flop the first few times, but if you are not altogether decrepit, you will presently be finishing on your feet as though it all were mere child's play.

As I mention in the chapter on breathing, sedentary persons who get too little general exercise, riding even when they could and should be walking, may have nearly a fourth of the entire volume of their blood stagnating in the splanchnic pool, that vast network of vessels in the greater, abdominal, body cavity and viscera. I believe somersaulting puts this slack blood back into circulation more effectively than any exercise you can take in so short a time.

In my files are scores of letters from men and women in their sixties and seventies who are Somersaultuaquans. The late Luther Burbank, I remember, appeared in the newsreels somersaulting on his lawn on the occasion of his 75th birthday.

As exercise, somersaults aren't much—I would say half a dozen, which you may do in less than half a minute, are equivalent to walking six to eight blocks on level ground. Still, I know of devotees who make them their complete day's exercise. Some even declare it is exercise effective for reducing. To prove it, here's a testimonial which I just can't help citing although, quite frankly, it seems to me preposterous:

> "Two months ago I weighed 304 pounds. I began turning somersaults as you suggested. Now I weight 250 pounds . . ."
> (Mrs. A.H.F.)

Personally I ascribe the lady's weight reduction to some cause or causes her letter fails to make clear. I am sure a brisk daily walk or other equivalent exercise is far more effective than mere somersaulting if reducing is what you are after. Besides, the main part of any reduction regimen is diet. Make of Mrs. A.H.F.'s statement what you will.

Novices determined to start the practice should use a mat, mattress, pillow or padding of some kind for their first attempts. But an experienced roller requires only two square yards of level ground, lawn, carpet, rug or bare floor. I do my own morning rolls on the bedroom rug. Then, whenever I've been tied for long hours to my desk and an idea gets stuck in my subconscious or something irks me, I roll a few right beside my desk and presto, the idea comes unstuck and annoyances no longer pall.

Stagnation, or congestion, in the splanchnic pool is a common predisposing factor of hemorrhoids, both the internal or bleeding kind and the external, painful piles. It is also a predisposing factor of common pelvic disorders in both men and women.

Somersaultauquans testify that rolling has served as a remedy for a number of other conditions, among them poor circulation associated with sallow complexion and cold feet, intestinal stasis, flatulence, fullness and distress attributed to "gas," chloasma, which means moth patches or liver spots, "biliousness," the menstrual difficulties of young women and the hot flashes of the middle aged ones, periodic sick headache or migraine, and finally insomnia. If you are subject to any of these complaints, all I can say is that it can do you no harm to try somersaulting and see for yourself whether or not you are helped.

If you are rapidly turning into an old crock—that is, if for several years you have done nothing more than lie, sit, stand and occasionally walk a block or two—and now have developed a wild, harum-scarum notion to try rolling somersaults, do it in the privacy of your own bedroom. I also suggest that you not only use a couple of mattresses at first but also shed hair pins, girdle, corset, bustle, cud of tobacco and false teeth. You might also take out a small accident policy before you try it.

From time to time somebody scolds me severely and even threatens to sue because the first time he or she tried to roll a somersault it brought on a sick or dizzy spell. All I can say about that is again to emphasize that I do not prescribe somersaults for anybody. If you choose to roll them, you must do so at your own peril.

But I do happen to think that for industrial and domestic slaves who cannot afford to indulge in expensive daily diversions such as a game of golf, tennis, baseball, basketball, bowls or other exercise, a few dozen somersaults, which will take only a few seconds, will serve as a partial substitute and a fine morale builder.

Chapter Thirteen

CALL IT CRI:
COMMON RESPIRATORY
INFECTIONS

A survey of both urban and rural areas in various parts of the country made by the Public Health Service some years ago indicated that three-fourths of the everyday work of doctors is the diagnosis and treatment of the common respiratory infections and their complications and consequences.

Just what are the common respiratory infections?

They are acute illnesses or diseases which spread from person to person mainly via droplet infection, that is to say, the germ or virus of the disease is carried in moisture droplets either in the visible and palpable or invisibly and impalpably fine spray given off when we cough, sneeze or talk.

The common respiratory infections have in common (1) the fact that in all of them the infective agent enters the body through the lining of nose or throat and (2) they are all spread to other persons mainly, as already stated, via cough, sneeze or conversation spray. This spray has a range of ten or 12 feet in open-face coughing or sneezing, two to five feet in ordinary conversation.

Here are the more familiar respiratory infections:

Coryza
Acute pharyngitis (sore throat)

Acute tonsillitis
Quinsy
Diphtheria
Scarlet fever
Measles
Mumps
German measles
Whooping cough
Influenza
Poliomyelitis (infantile paralysis)
Cerebro-spinal meningitis
Septic sore throat
Chicken pox
Smallpox
Encephalitis
Pneumonia
Pulmonary tuberculosis.

To list a disease as respiratory is not to imply that the disease may not sometimes be spread in another way—as by kissing or via unwashed or insufficiently washed eating or drinking utensils.

The old-timers assumed that chicken pox and smallpox were contagious, that is, spread by contact. I have not been able to form an opinion on that, but public health authorities agree that the infective agent in both diseases is a filtrable virus given off from mouth, nose or throat and transmitted to other persons in moisture droplets of cough, sneeze or conversation spray, just as measles, diphtheria or scarlet fever is.

Another thing respiratory infections have in common is their prodromal symptoms, which are so much alike that it is difficult to tell in the early hours of the illness just what the patient may be coming down with.

Of course this is no problem for the ninnyhammer. He assures his friends and associates it's just a bad "cold" so they needn't worry about getting peppered by his conversation spray. When or if they do get peppered, the poor ginks will blame it on some change of weather, wet feet or what have you. Thus, a stinker can share whatever he happens to have with every unwary person who happens to be within conversational spray range, and no one will censure him for it.

THE GOLDEN RULE OF HYGIENE   All of the common respiratory infections are most communicable in the early hours of the illness, before it is possible to tell which it is going to be. So the only fair thing to do is to isolate yourself or wear a suitable mask from the very beginning of the indisposition, to prevent spread of the infection. We'll explain later what constitutes a suitable mask.

Now I submit that if you can't tell in the early hours or maybe the first day or two what it is that ails you, you should call it *c r i* until the diagnosis is made. C r i (pronounced Kree), a coined word, is an abbreviation of the cumbersome term *common respiratory infection*.

Call it *c r i* if you are a nice, kind person.

Call it "cold" if you're a bit of a stinker.

When you call the indisposition *c r i* you acknowledge and give fair warning that it is probably communicable. If a practicing physician strings patients along with the phony diagnosis "just a bad cold," his license should be revoked.

ALL IS NOT COLD THAT SHIVERS   Every one of the illnesses mentioned in the list may pass as "just a cold" at the onset, if you are ignorant or obstinate about it. It wouldn't matter if you persist in that delusion for as long as your illness lasts *provided* others do not share your delusion and, consequently, share whatever infection you may happen to have.

The reason why all honest folk should discard the term "cold" as a label and adopt the term "cri" instead is now obvious. Even if you yourself don't care whether or not you have a communicable disease, it is only decent and fair to give others who come within range a break, to warn them of the risk that they may catch whatever you're coming down with. If you say, "I think I've got a little cold," you are trying to disarm people; if, on the other hand, you say, "I suppose it's the cri," you are giving every one fair warning to keep his distance.

That brings us to the question of the Golden Rule of Hygiene. If you're a good citizen you know what you should do. If you're a scoundrel you can get away with murder under the name of "the common cold" and have plenty of "scientific" or at least politically prominent testimony to support your malicious conduct. As long as the majority of people believe there is such an illness as a "cold" due to change of weather or some trifling dampness, draft or similar "exposure" (a quaint notion still sanctioned by certain politicians appointed health commissioners), viciously ignorant persons will continue to spread their respiratory infections indiscriminately.

When we adopt the name "cri," pending diagnosis of the specific nature of an illness, that does not imply that it is necessarily infectious (due to germs invading body tissues), nor communicable. It means merely that while we don't yet know what the trouble is, the chances are it is one or another of the common respiratory infections mentioned in the list.

Coryza, for instance, is most frequently an acute infection, and the stuffy and running nose, the sneezing, red eyes and general wretchedness of the trouble lasts several days. But we know that a condition hard for the layman to distinguish from typical coryza may be caused by (a) hay fever; (b) hyperesthetic rhinitis or individual sensitivity to some foreign protein (a state akin to asthma in origin); (c) by-effects of certain medicines in persons with idiosyncrasy, notably iodides, quinine and aspirin; (d) mechanical variations in general circulation from casual environmental changes in persons who are subject to chronic lesions of the upper respiratory tract, such as chronic rhinitis (catarrh), thickened turbinates, chronic sinusitis, adenoids, chronic middle ear inflammation. A peculiarity of all these non-infectious types of coryza ("head cold" to you) is that the attack is abrupt, the nose beginning to run or the victim beginning to sneeze or cough or feel uncomfortable or chilly as soon as he is "exposed" or imagines he is "exposed" to draft, dampness or cold. And the attack passes off as abruptly as it began.

Please do not lose sight of the fact that no one, be he physician, health expert or plain layman, can define or identify a "cold." So far as we know, there is no specific illness or ailment for which "cold" is a precise name. Nor is there a specific illness or ailment for which "cri" is a precise name. What "cri" stands for is any acute respiratory infection you may have, until or unless the nature of the trouble becomes manifest. So you see, I hope, how much difference it makes whether you elect to think or say you have a "common cold" or to assume you have the "cri."

I could fill a large book with the testimony of all kinds of people who have told me of their experiences, but after all, "he that complies against his will is of his own opinion still." I'll quote only the view of Vilhjalmur Stefansson, the famous Arctic explorer who lived five years in the Arctic, though other polar explorers believed a white man could not subsist on the food obtainable there the year around.

Mr. Stefansson describes in his book, *The Friendly Arctic,* many experiences which make our ordinary notions of "exposure" seem insignificant: day after day of wading through ice water, travel over ice and snow in weather that froze noses, fingers, cheeks. Yet here is what he says in a private communication: "No one in any of our parties has ever, so far as I know, suffered the slightest ill effect from indefinite exposure to damp . . . Seldom a day when the feet of all the Indians we were with were not wet all day. I had Eskimo footwear and my feet were never wet while I was with the Indians, but I do not remember that there was any difference between us as to catching cold. This occurred when we met strangers and not when we happened to get wet. I don't want to pretend deciding anything, but certainly all my evidence, whether from experience or observation, is completely negative. I have never seen any connection between wet feet and head colds."

I suppose some of our politically prominent health authorities in Yankeeland would tip back in their swivel chairs, plump their oxford shod feet on the radiator and dictate bulletins dismissing such evidence as trivial and warning the simple public against stray zephyrs or dew—didn't George Washington get some snow on his coat collar shortly before he succumbed to diphtheria, angina, quinsy, edema of the larynx or whatever made them bleed the man to death?

SHORT COURSE IN PHYSIOLOGY   If you are unaccustomed to strenuous exertion you are likely to get soreness and stiffness in the muscles the day after a violent effort or a hard game unless you take care to prevent too sudden cooling after the exercise. The better trained, the more accustomed to sustained muscular exertion, the less likely you are to suffer such lameness.

This is not due, as many people imagine, to suppression of sweat. Sweat, as I have said before, is practically nothing but water and common salt; any waste matter, excretion or "poison" present in the sweat is insignificant. Do not be misled by the specious suggestions of charlatans. Soreness is due entirely to retention, in and about the muscles, of products of combustion: the hard work done by the muscles is actually greatly increased oxidation or combustion of fuel, or blood sugar, within the muscles, and that produces the overheating of body and blood, which in turn brings about increased sweating which is the natural means of cooling the body. These combustion products, principally carbonic acid and lactic acid, are in ordinary circumstances carried away *through the circulation* as fast as they accumulate but during an extraordinary effort they accumulate faster than the circulation can remove them; and so, if circulation is suddenly *decreased* by the action of cold on the surface at a time when the muscles and other tissues are fairly choked with their own combustion products, muscular soreness and disability is the inevitable consequence.

Note that waste matter is removed through the veins: carbon dioxide, lactic acid and so on are carried to the lungs and kidneys to be excreted from the body; they are NOT to any appreciable degree thrown off through the sweat glands. If you fix this little lesson in physiology firmly in your mind it may save you time, money and health. You will know what to say when some quack seeks to sell you a glorified sweating course to "rid the system of waste matter or poisons." Remember, practically no poison or waste matter is eliminated or excreted in the sweat; only water and salt. Incidentally, mild exercise within three hours after a hard race is far superior to any kind of rubdown or passive exercise or massage to prevent or relieve muscular stiffness.

In my opinion the use of bacterin—or "bacterial vaccine, serum, inoculation," as it is variously called by the uninitiated—has not proved effective in immunizing against cri. In certain cases of frequent recurrence, however, a bacterin of autogenous source—that is, prepared from a culture from the lesion in the individual case— is sometimes of marked value.

I offer these suggestions merely as my personal views and for whatever they may be worth to you. Since three-fourths of the daily work of physicians is attributable to respiratory infection and subsequent complications (including much throat, nose, ear and chest surgery), I assure you I weigh with an earnest sense of responsibility everything I teach or suggest in reference to the question.

One honest old physician disposed of curbstone consultations by telling people who asked what he used for a cold, that he used two dozen soft linen handkerchiefs. Yet a single "ethical" medicine manufacturer, who supplies physicians but does not offer his wares to the public, lists no less than 150 products which according to his catalog are "indicated" in the treatment of "common cold." A manufacturer of a popular nostrum recently paid stockholders $6,000,-000 in four years, and showed $3,704,606 net profits in one year! People who recover in a fortnight like to give testimonials. And people who believe in the "common cold" haven't much faith in the doctor who has no specific remedy or treatment for it!

I BELIEVE IN PREVENTION   Now I shall offer some positive ideas or suggestions bearing upon immunity and prevention of the cri. These are my own ideas and teachings—I do not know whether a majority of physicians share these beliefs. You may accept them or reject them, as you wish.

Any one who wears more clothing than is necessary for physical comfort is likely to have insufficient immunity against respiratory infections.

The custom or habit of overheating dwellings, shops and offices, churches, theaters, public conveyances, likewise interferes with or retards development or maintenance of the individual's optimum normal immunity.

The influence of the ultraviolet in sunlight or in skyshine (indirect or diffused light) on naked skin is essential for full development of immunity. Perhaps this influence is the mysterious factor which makes "fresh air" healthful and "bad," "foul" or vitiated air unhealthful, though of course we know that movement of the air and the amount of moisture it contains are the chief factors determining comfort or discomfort of the air. In all circumstances I should advise every one, young or old, healthy or invalid, to expose as much

of the skin area as possible to as much sunlight or daylight as may
be available or endurable short of sunburn or frostbite. With Ben
Franklin I believe a morning "air bath," even in the privacy of
one's bedroom, is an excellent habit. I advocate nudity in private,
not public nudism. Finally, I advise parents to encourage the
natural desire of a child to go barefoot or with knees or legs bare,
in any kind of weather, provided the child enjoys it and is not
mentally defective.

So far we have said nothing at all about ultraviolet light from
artificial sources. The mercury-vapor quartz lamp, the carbon arc
lamp and some other lamps do deliver ultraviolet rays, though in
small quantity or proportion compared with the quantity or proportion of ultraviolet rays in noonday sunlight in clear weather. I
can recommend no particular ultraviolet lamp. If you contemplate
renting or buying one you should inquire of your physician as to its
efficiency. All I can say is that ultraviolet rays from a lamp are
the same in effect as ultraviolet rays from the sun, though far inferior in quantity per square inch of skin surface. However, unskilled application of ultraviolet rays from such a lamp may cause
a burn; sometimes serious sunburn.

In my opinion no specific diet either prevents or cures or "breaks
up" cri, although the adequacy of the diet in providing the essential
vitamins to maintain good general nutrition may be important, as
will appear presently.

The diet of children and young people almost universally provides insufficient thiamin, riboflavin and vitamin D, calcium, phosphorus and iodine. Therefore, I urge that young people, especially
in the late autumn, winter and early spring season, should have as
a regular supplement for the diet six Ray-D tablets—all may be
eaten with a single meal, or two may be taken with each of the
three meals daily. Ray-D tablets (Neoco) contain fair amounts of
these essentials.

Vitamin A has been exploited, mainly by manufacturers of
proprietary products, as an agent which "helps" prevent "colds."
Whenever the vendor uses the trick word "helps" in proclaiming
the efficacy of his nostrum it is well to remember he does so in
order to satisfy the annoying requirements imposed by government
authorities such as the Food and Drug Administration and that the

product is probably not worth a damn for the prevention of any ailment.

But vitamin A serves a specific purpose or function in nutrition which, in my opinion, warrants the belief that it is essential in the development and maintenance of the highest degree of immunity against respiratory infections in general. It promotes the integrity or healthiness of the mucous membranes lining the respiratory tract. Normal condition and functioning of the mucous membranes constitutes a first line of defense against invading bacteria. Therefore, particularly for young persons who show a tendency toward adenoids, enlarged tonsils and frequent or constant snuffles, perhaps with enlarged lymph nodes or "kernels" in the neck, I recommend an optimal daily ration of natural vitamin A, that is, considerably more vitamin A than you are likely to get in any diet. An optimal daily ration is assured if you take with breakfast a tablet of Nion nio-a-lets which contains 25,000 international units of vitamin A.

I must mention here that a difference exists between natural vitamin A and carotene, or provitamin A. Vitamin A is ready to be absorbed by the body whereas carotene or provitamin A requires conversion into vitamin A by metabolism. It is therefore less efficient than natural vitamin A. This distinction is often overlooked.

Foods richest in natural vitamin A are milk, cream, butter, cheese, egg yolk, mammalian liver; foods richest in carotene (or provitamin A which requires conversion into vitamin A), are apricots, fresh, frozen or dried, string beans, broccoli, carrots, chard, escarole (also known as endive and French chicory greens—having curly leaves), kale, lettuce, fresh green peas, spinach, sweet potato, ripe banana, parsley, summer squash, orange or orange juice, tomato or tomato juice, fresh or canned, dried prunes, canned salmon, yellow peaches, cherries, nectarines, cantaloupe, turnip greens, beet greens, dandelion greens, and dried powdered grass when it shall become available.

It is possible, though difficult nowadays, to get an optimal daily ration of vitamin A, that is, more than is necessary merely to prevent such deficiency manifestations as nightblindness, dry eyes and toadskin, from the diet alone if a sufficient quantity and variety of the foods mentioned be consumed daily. Even so, it would not be easy to get 25,000 international units a day that way. That's what Nion Vitamin A Acetate gives in a single tablet. One tablet daily for infant, child or adult.

Dr. Leonard Hill, noted English physiologist and authority on ventilation and fresh air, dealt a great blow to the powerful interests that promote coddling in England and in America when he declared that "It is absurd to put on an overcoat when going out for a walk. It is good to go out and be braced by feeling cold and so be impelled to take vigorous exercise." I gather it is still being done in England, but here in America nobody walks except the mailman and a few tramps who are not going anywhere and are in no great hurry to arrive.

Clothing of any kind that is not necessary for protection against excessive cold or wet or heat or sunlight is detrimental to health. It impairs the heat-regulating functions of the skin. It excludes light.

We have always associated a coat of tan with health and vigor; and whiteness or pallor with weakness or sickness. Now we begin to understand why. The pigment in the skin is produced by exposure to sun and air; it is a kind of dynamic accumulator. It receives, stores and serves out to the body as needed some element or factor essential in the utilization of vitamins, especially those vitamins concerned in immunity against infection.

In many homes it is, and certainly should be, the rule that any member of the household with the c r i shall isolate himself behind a suitable mask to protect other members against infection.

THE HAZARD OF CONVERSATIONAL SPRAY Everybody knows it is extremely unpleasant if not dangerous to be coughed or sneezed upon. The intelligentsia are vaguely aware that the mouth, throat or nose secretions that are shot forth by a cough or sneeze, are likely to carry infection directly to the victim. Even a few politicians holding berths as health commissioners from time to time publish bulletins warning the public to beware of the open-face cough or sneeze in time of epidemic. Don't ever make me king of this country or even elect me to the senate, for one of the first laws I would make would be to provide a suitable reward for any citizen who barks his knuckles on the jaws of the boor who thus spits on anyone within his spray range.

The vital thing which many educated people do *not* know is that this moisture spray given off in coughing or sneezing and effectively stopped by holding hand or handkerchief over nose and mouth, is likewise given off in ordinary conversation and not even guarded against, for the very reason that people do not know the facts about it.

For the life of me I can't see why people who can accept being informed of the peril in cough or sneeze spray should be so squeamish about hearing of the danger in conversational spray. Yet the commercial interests that control popular education in Yankeeland forbid instruction of the public about this, at least via radio. In a series of health talks I gave over a national radio chain I was permitted to refer briefly to the hazard of the uncovered cough or sneeze, but the broadcasting censor saw to it that I made no allusion whatsoever to conversational spray. The great nostrum makers couldn't sell their wares so easily if the public were not so ill-informed.

Practically the only difference between sneeze or cough spray and conversation spray is the range of the spray.

By precise scientific measurements it has been determined that sneeze or cough spray (both visible spray and that composed of invisible fine droplets) carries from ten to 12 feet. The spray given off from nose and mouth in ordinary conversation, mostly composed in invisibly fine droplets, carries less than five, usually two or three feet.

It is in the droplets of the spray that infection is carried. I believe this is practically the only way respiratory infection occurs. Of course the act of kissing might transfer such infection, but practically all cri may be ascribed to spray infection, and now that even the unenlightened portion of the population is beginning to comprehend that it is not good for your health to be spit upon, I hope to make some of the intelligentsia aware of conversational spray infection and how to avoid it.

YOU GET SPRAYED AS YOU SHAKE HANDS Here it is well to mention the theory that the custom of shaking hands may be a mode of infection. I doubt that hand shaking spreads disease, because we know the specific germs of such disease as influenza, diphtheria, meningitis, pneumonia quickly lose their virulence or power to cause disease, if they do not merely die on exposure to air, light, dryness or a temperature below that of the blood.

I do not believe that objects or furniture contaminated by cough, sneeze or conversational spray of a person with infectious disease are likely to be a source of infection to any one. It is my firm conviction that only the spray you catch on the fly, so to speak, and take directly into nose or mouth, can harm you.

Knowing the range of cough or sneeze spray and that of conversational spray, you can contrive to keep out of range and thus avoid many such infections. Or if the requirements of business or work render it impossible to keep beyond the four-foot range, then often you can take advantage of a screen which will effectually stop the spray—such as a glass partition or panel between the window clerk and the patron. No disease is carried through or by the air, and no disease germs are present in the air expired in ordinary breathing. In the best contagious disease hospitals low partitions or screens are all that separate the patients from each other, or the convalescents from visitors. There is no attempt to prevent germs from floating in the air because we know germs do not get about that way. Germs can travel only when and where they may be carried; they cannot move a fraction of an inch themselves.

A person interviewing or meeting a constant succession of clients should arrange desk, chairs, counter or table with a view to insuring a five-foot space between faces.

During the great "flu" epidemic many persons wore masks—not such a bad idea, either. It would be more effective if every person with cri wore such a mask. It should be made of not less than 10 layers of gauze or cheesecloth having not less than 32 threads to the inch, cover nose and mouth, and be tied in place by tapes over the head and behind the neck, or attached to spectacle frames. It is necessary to have several such masks and change two or three times a day. Ordinary washing with soap and water and ironing sufficiently sterilizes the mask. Of course the mask merely catches the moisture droplets of the spray; it would hardly filter out germs.

Super-speed photographs of sneeze spray widely printed in

newspapers and magazines have impressed many readers, but unfortunately no pictures of the spray produced by conversation were published. The technologists who made the pictures estimated that the droplets, laden with germs, travel at the rate of 150 feet a second and they imagined some of the droplets might float about for a considerable time, to deposit their loads of bacteria upon the mucous membrane of the person who might eventually inhale them.

I believe there is no serious danger from that. I believe any disease germs contained in such moisture droplets are practically certain to die or at least lose their virulence or capacity to do harm if they are exposed for more than a second to drying, light, cold, as in floating about an ordinary room for a second or two. I believe the only mouth spray that is at all dangerous is that which travels directly from one person to another. In other words, a direct hit is essential for infection. This may happen at a distance of ten or 12 feet in sneezing or coughing, but not more than five feet in conversation.

THE SILVERS' MASK   A mask which is more practical and more comfortable for those rendering personal service—physicians or specialists or nurses examining or treating nose and throat patients, oculists, optometrists and opticians examining eyes or adjusting glasses, dentists, barbers, hair dressers—is the one devised by Dr. Lewis J. Silvers of New York, noted exponent of diathermy extirpation of the tonsils. The mask is made of a 9" x 7" piece of washed X-ray safety film or firm cellophane with corners well rounded off, snap fasteners inserted one and a half inches from the upper corners by means of which the mask may be snapped in place on headband (or head mirror or lamp worn by a doctor, on a plain headband if the worker does not require mirror or lamp). The mask is perfectly transparent and stands away from contact with the face for ventilation and comfort.

For tellers, ticket sellers, cashiers and others who serve many people daily, the most satisfactory mask or screen is a glass window, with an opening well below face level through which money, checks or change may be passed. So far as contamination of money, check, paper or metal is concerned, again you need have no anxiety—it is only the direct hit that matters.

Chapter Fourteen

WHAT TO DO ABOUT CRI

Without a "cold cure" or sure fire method of "breaking it up" how can you best cope with an attack of the cri?

First let me mention some things to avoid.

Never take a nostrum that purports to be good for colds, grippe, and other troubles. There are scores of them all containing injurious coaltar derivatives such as acetanilid, phenacetin, antipyrin, or aspirin or similar pain-killer, nerve-deadener or fever-reducer. Such drugs produce their analgesic effects at the expense of the natural means of self-defense, let us say.

Personally, I should prefer the ordinary discomforts of any such mild indisposition of a headache or tolerable pain in the neck than resort to dope that tends to break down red blood corpuscles, damage the integrity of the heart and interfere with the oxygen-carrying function of hemoglobin. I might chance one dose of five to ten grains of aspirin or if I were in great pain and could not reach a physician I might even take a second dose of this least dangerous of pain-killers; but I'd hesitate to do so in just any circumstances, and believe me, I'd remain quietly in bed or at rest while under the influence of any such medicine. To my mind the fool who takes such dope and keeps up and about is courting disaster.

HOT MUSTARD FOOT BATH In any attack of cri accompanied by chilly sensations or feverishness or evidence of congestion of the tissues, a hot mustard foot bath is always good treatment. The foot tub or bucket should contain water as hot as the feet will bear, up half way to the knees, with a small handful of mustard flour or powder mixed in. The foot bath is best given by a nurse to the patient tucked between blankets in bed, but if you get the bed all ready, with hot bottle at the foot and light warm covers and blankets arranged, you can take the bath sitting wrapped in a blanket, not night clothes. Soak the feet in the bath 15 to 30 minutes, with hotter water added as often as necessary to keep the bath so hot the feet can only barely endure it. Meanwhile you should have all the hot lemonade, or any other hot beverage, water, milk, tea, soup, you care to take. After the bath, lie well covered for an hour or two before removing the sweaty covers and putting on dry ones.

Please understand clearly that while any sudden chilling may defeat the purpose of the h.m.f.b., which is essentially to equalize circulation and relieve congestion, there is absolutely no danger in sudden suppression of sweating so induced—sweat being a purely mechanical reaction to the heat, a natural means of cooling the body or regulating temperature.

LAXATIVES I myself must have a pretty serious threat or scare before I'll consent to take a saline laxative or cathartic for cri. But if I get too anxious or if my general manager takes matters into her own hands and insists that I do something, I placate all hands by taking half a bottle or if necessary a whole bottle of freshly prepared solution of magnesium citrate. This is effervescing and when cold it is not at all unpleasant to take. A bottle holds 12 ounces, which is merely a moderate dose as salts go. If you should need it, see that the druggist prepares it on your order, and don't let him stick you with a bottle he has been keeping in readiness for days or weeks.

Diet is a minor matter. Fruits or their juices or any other beverages are all right if you like them. I take no stock in the prevailing hokum about "acidosis" and diet or medicine that opposes the hypothetical over-production of acid waste products. Neither do I accept the sweeping injunction to "feed a cold and starve a fever" —or is it vice versa?—as a sensible guide in therapy. If the patient is hungry of course he should take the nourishment he wants. If his appetite is poor, all right, probably it is better for him to skip a meal or two or to take only a bit of whatever he prefers.

The more liquid or fluid taken, the better. Have milk, buttermilk, soup, tea, coffee, cocoa, any fresh fruit juice or beverage and plenty of water, cold or hot, as preferred.

You may have noticed when you had coryza or sore throat that when you got snug in bed the trouble seemed alleviated. All the symptoms abate. Why? Because the circulation is equalized, there is more blood in the surface vessels, less in the congested or inflamed tissues. Similar condition is favored by (1) the hot mustard foot bath, (2) sleep, (3) belly breathing, and (4) staying in bed or going to bed even for a short nap, though a day in bed is universally recognized as the most effective way to cope with cri.

WHAT TO DO ABOUT THE CRI   So far as diagnosis and treatment are concerned it matters little whether you feel feverish or chilly, whether you stuff or starve it. The important thing is that you must:

(1) call it cri, since nobody knows what "cold" means. For that matter nobody knows what cri is in this stage of illness or indisposition, but you want to be fair so you call it cri, and so imply that you are probably coming down with one of the Common Respiratory Infections and want to give your friends a break. If you attempt to conceal the infectious character of the trouble under the disarming name "slight cold" you are playing a dirty trick on everyone who happens to come within your conversational spray range. So try to heed the golden rule of hygiene by calling it cri.

(2) Good citizen or scoundrel, it is your duty to keep out of school, church, shop, theatre, public conveyance or public gathering or meeting of any kind when you have such an illness—*before* it has been definitely diagnosed as something dangerous like diphtheria, infantile paralysis or influenza. If justice were done, the scoundrel who comes to school, church, the theater or afternoon tea while suffering with an alleged "slight cold" would be thrown out on his ear. People who break this rule sow the seeds of most of the illnesses physicians attend: grippe, pneumonia, sore throat, tonsillitis, measles and meningitis. All of these diseases masquerade

in the same way at onset and all are most communicable in the earliest stage, before the patient takes to bed.

(3) For the protection of those who must approach within your conversational spray range, wear a suitable mask over nose and mouth, as previously described.

(4) Keep your medicine, toilet and eating utensils separate and dispose of any nose or throat discharge by burning the paper handkerchiefs, precisely as though you knew your illness were diphtheria.

So far my instructions are mainly in the interest of public welfare. Due consideration for public welfare is an obligation in every case of cri, whether it turns out to be a trifling indisposition or a grave illness. No one can tell in the beginning just what it is going to be.

Please do not infer that the "common cold," either neglected or occurring when you happen to be run down or exhausted and so unable to "throw it off," may turn into a definite illness such as pneumonia. So far as physicians know, if the illness proves to be pneumonia, it was pneumonia from the very start. Anyone who suggests that any such transmutation can happen is only betraying his own ignorance. You may, however, aggravate your condition by being careless.

(5) In any case of cri it is generally beneficial to have a hot bath just before you go to bed, or better still a hot mustard foot bath in bed. The latter of course requires the services of a nurse. In either case it is advisable to remain in bed at least a day. Not, as I hope you won't assume, for fear of "taking more" of what ails you, but simply because in bed the circulation is equalized and congestion relieved. Everyone has noticed how the stuffed up nostrils clear and the misery and ache in the head lets up after you get into bed, warmed up and composed for sleep.

A hot mustard foot bath administered in bed is as good first aid treatment for acute earache, acute toothache with swelling or inflammation, acute bronchitis, acute pleurisy, acute pneumonia and acute laryngitis, as for acute coryza. It is beneficial whether it induces sweating or not. It relieves congestion by drawing blood to the surface. If sweating occurs it is simply an index of the efficiency of the treatment. The amount of "poison," waste matter or disease toxins that may be "thrown off" with even the most copious sweating is insignificant in any circumstances. There is no harm or danger in throwing off the covers and cooling off after such a bath, whether there is profuse sweating or none. Any patient old enough or with brains enough to know what is comfortable and what isn't should have his own way about this.

(6) If you are young and vigorous, drink all the cool or cold water or fruit juice (sweetened if you wish) you like. If you are old and not so vigorous take your liquid warm or hot, if you prefer. If you are neither young nor old, why, suit your taste about it. If you don't care for water, milk, soup or other wholesome beverage, why you needn't take a darn thing.

(7) The homely saying, "Feed a cold and starve a fever"—is misleading if taken seriously. It may be all right for a well nourished individual who remains in bed to skip a meal or even to fast for 24 hours; such a rest for metabolism may be distinctly beneficial in many instances. But it is a mistake to try fasting if you remain up and at work. Overeating and too hasty eating produces portal engorgement (congestion in liver area) and consequent overfulness of the vessels about the nasal passages, throat and sinuses. This is rather a predisposing or aggravating factor of the cri.

(8) In any case of cri where there is cough, tickling, dryness, soreness or hoarseness, prepare immediately and use every two hours as directed, Old Doc Brady's Fool Proof Cough Medicine. Detailed instructions will follow.

(9) The best counterirritant liniment or embrocation for infant, child or adult with any form of cri, in my judgment, is camphor liniment, commonly called camphorated oil. This should be freshly made by dissolving an ounce of camphor in coarse powder form in four ounces of warm cottonseed oil (USP) or olive oil (British P). A little may be rubbed over bridge of nose and over the throat and the chest. In the case of young infants do not leave the clothing saturated or soiled with camphor liniment, for the baby may inhale a harmful quantity if left like that for hours.

(10) Most nostrums purporting to be "cold cures" or good for "grippe" and the like are practically nothing but acetanilide, phenacetine, antipyrin or one of the related coal tar analgesics or

pain-killers more or less disguised with other unimportant drugs. Without attempting to explain the harm and the danger involved in the use of these coal tar derivatives I'll say I believe the use of such drugs early in the illness is the straw that turns the scale against recovery in many instances. Certainly no blood-destroying, sense-deadening, heart-weakening drug has any remedial value in any illness, except to dull aches, pains, distress or weariness. So my opinion and advice is that if you have cri you should let such dope severely alone, and only when distress is unendurable seek relief in a dose of acetylsalicylic acid (aspirin to you). As a pain-killer, sense-deadener or analgesic, acetylsalicylic acid, in a dose of five to ten grains, repeated not more than once every two hours, is the least dangerous I know. I say least dangerous, not the safest, for it is by no means free from untoward effects. Like the more dangerous analgesics mentioned above, aspirin has no specific remedial effects so far as we can determine, aside from its pain-benumbing action.

(11) From general observation and experience I have concluded that the use of nose drops or medicaments inserted in the nostrils in any manner is inadvisable for children and may be dangerous for infants. Adults, however, sometimes find considerable relief from the use of drops, vapor, spray or balm or salve inserted or applied in the nasal passages.

(12) If any medicine under the sun deserves the name "cri cure" it is that old stand-by, quinine. We are bound to recognize that quinine holds general preference among physicians and laymen as a remedy for "checking" or "breaking up" the cri.

Three grains of quinine sulphate, in capsule or in sugar-coated or chocolate-coated pill or tablet every four hours for an adult, one grain every four hours for a child weighing less than 50 pounds, has proved the most satisfactory self-treatment or home treatment for so-called grippe, flu or cri or any common respiratory infection in the early stage before even a doctor can tell just what is developing.

Attempts to explain scientifically how quinine works in the prevention and treatment of the all too common respiratory infections are not very satisfactory. For that matter there is no satisfactory scientific explanation for the prophylactic and remedial value of quinine against malaria. Certainly it is not due to any germicidal or plasmodicidal power in quinine itself—at least it exerts no such power when mixed in comparable concentration with culture of cri germs or malaria plasmodia in the test tube. Nevertheless, I am thoroughly convinced that quinine aids in the body's defense and fight against pneumonia, acute bronchitis, flu, grippe, or whatever you call it before you can be certain what is developing.

It doesn't matter whether the quinine be taken in the form of quinine sulphate, quinine bi-sulphate, quinine hydrocholoride or quinine tannate (a form sometimes preferred for children, as it does not taste bad mixed in chocolates), or whether in tablet, pill, capsule, lozenge or solution.

As a prophylactic ration which means the dose advisable for building or maintaining good immunity in time of cri epidemic, I recommend two grains each night and morning for adults, one grain night and morning for children. This ration is best taken with or after breakfast and supper. It should be continued for several weeks, or until the epidemic is over.

CHILDREN ARE THE VICTIMS OF THE GREAT DELUSION
Children are the greatest sufferers from the too common "cold" delusion. Any one who has children or who loves children should give the question the most careful consideration. More than three-fourths of illness among children is directly or indirectly due to preventable respiratory infection.

I mention elsewhere that acute appendicitis is sometimes a consequence of cri. It is well recognized that acute appendicitis in children is not rarely a sequel to, or a complication of, repeated attacks of tonsillitis which on careful investigation are found to be due to Pneumococcus infection, the strain of germs commonly responsible for pneumonia. The same germ is found responsible for the appendicitis in these cases.

A few suggestions about the management of a child with the cri:

HYGIENE AT SCHOOL   First, it is the parent's duty to keep the child home from school and from contact with playmates or relatives whenever the child manifests any signs or symptoms of coryza, stuffy or runny nose, sore throat, hoarseness or cough.

Second, it is the teacher's duty to report immediately to the school physician any child who comes to school with such signs or symptoms. If the school is a backwoods institution or one in a town where the grafters steal the funds which should provide daily attendance and inspection by a physician, then the teacher or superintendent of the school owes it to the safety of the other children and to the reputation of the school to send home any such child and to refuse readmittance until the child comes with a physician's certificate or assurance that the trouble is not communicable or that the contagious period of the illness has passed.

The parents should see that the child developing cri is put to bed immediately and kept there until the trouble subsides or a physician takes charge of the case. Of course other members of the household must keep out of the child's range. Where young children are concerned, erect a barrier, a gate or rope which will keep the well child or children not less than six feet away from the patient. That is beyond conversational spray range. Of course if the child is too young to learn about the importance of covering mouth and nose with handkerchief whenever it is necessary to sneeze or cough, other children are endangered if they enter the same room.

Either the patient or those who must come into close contact or association can best guard against communication of cri by wearing a mask.

A physician I know who treats nose and throat diseases suffered several serious infections from being coughed on, and finally devised a protective mask to wear when he is treating patients whose trouble is infectious. He attached to the frame of his headlamp a piece of clear washed X-ray film which serves as an effective barrier.

Young children are likely to cough excessively and with a croupy sound when they have a mild coryza, especially soon after going to bed. Perhaps if the child can be made to sleep in a semi-prone position, that is, more nearly face down, or quite prone with the face turned toward the side and the head resting on a very low pillow, this harsh and useless coughing may be prevented. It is due largely to mucous secretion trickling back from the nasal passages down into the throat.

Coryza in a nursing infant is a serious handicap and demands the attendance of the physician.

Where there is much irritation of the throat, hoarseness and cough, considerable relief may be obtained by inhaling for several minutes the steam or vapor given off from a pitcher or can of water containing a teaspoonful of compound tincture of benzoin, the benzoin being put in the boiling water and the steam inhaled through a paper cone or a towel over the pitcher. This may be repeated every hour or two if it affords relief.

A cold wet compress—that is, a cloth or small towel wrung out of ice cold water—applied to the front and sides of neck—and covered with dry flannel, becomes a warm compress in a short time and has a soothing effect on any acute congestion or irritation in the throat, larynx or windpipe.

TECHNIQUE OF BLOWING THE NOSE   There is a right way to blow the nose and several wrong ways.

The right way to do it is this:

First, always bend the head forward so that you are looking down toward the floor before you blow.

Second, never pinch the nostrils nor hold the handkerchief or paper in contact with the nose, but instead hold it an inch or two below the nose while blowing.

Never close the mouth, but keep it wide open while blowing the nose.

Never blow forcibly, but only gently and steadily, the idea being not to force secretion from the nostrils but simply to favor drainage.

Pinching the nostrils, closing the mouth, holding the head erect and blowing forcibly may not only congest the middle ear or one or more sinuses but actually force the infection into one of these accessory cavities and cause acute otitis media, mastoiditis or sinusitis.

In general, the less the nose is blown the better. And the more gently or easily it is blown the better.

FOOLPROOF COUGH MEDICINE   In cases of cri characterized by cough or dryness and soreness or hoarseness the misinformed layman generally hankers after cough medicine. With rare exceptions the countless concoctions which purport to be good for cough depend on narcotic ingredients for their effect, which is merely to suppress the desire to cough by benumbing the senses for a while. In most instances this is foolish and dangerous, for ill-advised use of such "sedatives" turns the scale againt recovery in a good many cases. Besides choking off the impulse to cough the nostrum, whether of low degree or prescribed originally by a physician, lowers all the secretions and all the vital processes, and that's why such medicine retards or prevents prompt recovery. Particularly vicious is the practice of feeding such narcotic-laden "cough" medicine to children who cough with little cause or provocation. I have seen more than one infant done to death by morphine in cough medicine given by ignorant parents on the assurance of the corner druggist that the medicine was "perfectly harmless"—in spite of the warning printed on the label.

Since people set such store by "keeping the liver and bowels active" in the management of any such illness it is ridiculous how they resort to all kinds of physics for that purpose, yet dope themselves with other drugs which lessen all the secretions of the body.

Instead of attempting to choke off the impulse to cough when there's something the matter, wouldn't it be wiser to aid that function, and at the same time promote all the secretions or at least not retard them without reason? I think so, but of course I'm only a common ordinary doctor not bound by the tenets of any "school," cult or -pathy, and neither retained by any commercial interest nor bemused by any fad. From years of experience in practice and from long study and observation I have evolved a homely recipe which I offer as a foolproof cough medicine. It doesn't cure anything. On the other hand it will never kill anybody. It is suitable for the baby or yourself or gran'ma.

MAKE YOUR OWN COUGH MEDICINE   Steep or boil for 20 to 30 minutes a heaping teaspoonful of whole flaxseeds in a pint of water. Then dissolve in the flaxseed tea one ounce of citrate of soda and one ounce of glycerin, then add the juice of one lemon and finally three or four drops of peppermint (essence or oil of peppermint, or other flavor essence if you prefer). Strain the pint of medicine. The dose is a tablespoonful every two hours for two or three days; for a baby or young child a teaspoonful every two hours for a day or two. This is a gentle diuretic (promotes kidney secretion), a diaphoretic (promotes sweating), and a mildly sedative expectorant which tends to loosen, liquefy and ease coughing. Besides the medicine serves as an alkali to oppose any acidosis attending the illness.

Sodium citrate is an old standby. It was formerly much used as an addition to the baby's bottle where an alkali was desired to prevent coarse curdling of milk.

No serious harm is done if by mistake you drink the whole pint of foolproof cough medicine at a single dose—it would only act as a purgative.

I seriously recommend this medicine in any case of acute cri attended with soreness, rawness, hoarseness or huskiness and cough. I do not advise it for chronic cases, and I do not think it is of value for more than a day or two. This is the only medicine I consider worth while when I have the cri. But I'm funny that way. So don't mind me if you know more about these things than a simple practitioner like myself.

If there is any sore throat or any occasion to use a gargle or mouthwash, a solution of a heaping teaspoonful of boric acid in a pint of boiled water, used hot or cold, is at least as efficacious as any "antiseptic" you can buy for the purpose. The same solution, at about body temperature, is the most suitable as a nasal spray or for irrigating the nasal passages in any case where a mild antiseptic solution is required.

Finally it is simple discretion and good economy, when any cri is not clearly on the mend after the first twenty-four hours, to summon medical aid.

For preventing hoarseness or roughness of the voice, singers and speakers find the frequent use of a gargle in the course of a program or even just before singing or speaking helpful. The gargle consists of:

> Powdered alum .... rounded teaspoonful
> Barley Water .... one and a half cupfuls
> Mel Rosae (honey flavored with rose extract) ....
> ...... enough to fill half pint vial

Singers and speakers have used for years an agreeable yet efficacious astringent gargle originated by Mr. Joseph W. England, pharmacist in Philadelphia Hospital. It is prepared by dissolving two drams (two teaspoonfuls) of potassium chlorate in four ounces of boiling water, which stands cooling while one dram (one teaspoonful) of alum is dissolved in two and a half ounces of stronger rose water, to which are then added in the order named one-half ounce (tablespoonful) of glycerin, one-half ounce of plain syrup or honey (tablespoonful) and finally three drams (three teaspoonfuls) of fluid extract of eucalyptus rostrata (red gum). Shake up this ruby-red liquid and add it to the reserved portion. The product should be a clear ruby-red liquid of agreeable odor and taste. For use, add a tablespoonful of it to an equal quantity of water and gargle. Gargle once or twice within the half hour before singing or speaking. Or use it every few hours for relief of mild sore throat.

If the druggist cannot supply fluid extract or eucalyptus rostrata, fluid extract of kino may be substituted in the formula, using TWO drams (two teaspoonfuls) of it instead of three drams of red gum.

SPEAKING OF GARGLING   Precise scientific tests indicate that medicine applied in the form of a gargle scarcely gets beyond the front or oral entrance to the throat anyway. So far as remedial or curative treatment of tonsil, adenoid, or pharyngeal (throat) inflammations may be concerned, gargling is of questionable value; indeed, in acute inflammations it may be harmful. In mild or chronic conditions, if the use of a gargle gives any appreciable relief to discomfort, hoarseness or huskiness, it is unobjectionable. In general, gargling with antiseptic or germicidal agents may be altruistic, in that it tends to prevent spread of the throat infections to other persons.

But it is wasteful and rather futile so far as treatment of the trouble is concerned. Of course, the germs that are causing the trouble are in the tissues, not on the surface of the mucous membrane, and so no medicament applied to the surface can affect them at all.

Chapter Fifteen

A-HUM ON THE OLD CATARRH

Formerly *catarrh* meant inflammation of any mucous membrane. Mucous membrane lines every body cavity or opening that communicates with the outside world. More recently catarrh has signified particularly the inflammation of the mucous membrane lining the nasal passages, or chronic rhinitis.

Causes of simple chronic rhinitis are (1) living in an overheated, excessively dried out atmosphere indoors most of the time; (2) overeating—too large proportions of the calories yielded by pure starches and sugars, deficient in minerals and vitamins which have been removed or destroyed in process of refining natural food; (3) sedentary habit and the poor circulation accompanying it; (4) damage done by frequent infection; (5) habit of wearing excessive clothing.

CHRONIC RHINITIS   In simple nasal "catarrh" there is a long-standing low grade inflammation of the mucous membrane lining the nasal passages, with relaxed, flabby, boggy, congested, stuffy condition, now one side, now the other being swollen and nearly closed. Chronic rhinitis is annoying but does not affect general health. Persons who have it seem more susceptible to the cri than normal persons. Moreover individuals with chronic rhinitis react excessively to every trifling draft, change of temperature, change of clothing, variation of temperature and humidity indoors. They develop sudden stuffiness, perhaps running at the nose, sneezing or

146

coughing—and they insist this is proof that one "takes cold" from such "exposure," although the unpleasant symptoms last only as long as the exposure itself, disappearing as soon as the customary environment is restored. Their obstinacy is innocent however, for few subjects of chronic rhinitis ever have a full medical examination of the nose cavity made, and so they do not know what ails them. They imagine, usually becoming insistent if you try to reason with them, that hardened individuals may not be sensitive to drafts and the like but they are of finer nature and certainly do take cold if they even walk on damp pavements with their rubbers on.

Since few subjects of simple chronic rhinitis undergo proper medical examination, few ever seek treatment.

Aside from correction of bad hygiene—overheated rooms, excessive dryness of the heated air in homes and other buildings lacking air-conditioning, the habit of wearing more clothing than comfort demands, and overeating—the treatment of simple chronic rhinitis or "catarrh" is mainly topical, that is, by means of local application of suitable remedies to the nasal mucous membrane. Probably the most effective of these is an iodine-glycerine solution applied two or three times weekly by the physician—it is too strong for the patient to attempt to apply. This is not comfortable treatment—more or less burning, irritation and aching for half an hour must be expected following applications.

Another local application which the patient may use every day is precipitated sulphur. This is insufflated or blown into each nasal passage with a powder-blower once daily. It checks excessive secretion, heals excoriation, stops crust formation, prevents odor. Applied daily or each alternate day it is not unpleasant to use.

For regular daily spraying, douching or irrigating to clear the nasal passages of excessive secretion the standard Alkaline Antiseptic Solution, complete formula for which is given in every drugstore's National Formulary, may be used; or a simple solution of boric acid in water will serve the purpose. Either of these is well suited for home use as mouthwash, gargle or nasal spray or irrigation. The solution should always be comfortably warm for use in the nose.

In using Alkaline Antiseptic Solution, dilute it with three or four times as much water as solution in the atomizer, use a straight tip spray, direct the spray horizontally along the floor of the nasal cavity with head held erect. If boric acid solution is used, the right strength is a rounded teaspoonful of boric acid dissolved in a pint of boiled water. This too should be warmed to about body warmth for use in the nose, eyes, ears or as a gargle.

By the way, persons subject to nasal allergy, manifested as hyperesthetic rhinitis, hay fever or similar symptoms, sudden profuse watering at the nose, sneezing on slight provocation or temperamental stuffiness of the breathing passages, will find potassium chloride efficacious and harmless for symptomatic relief. It doesn't cure anything, merely gives relief just as adrenalin might do—two Kalion tablets taken in a glassful of water whenever needed, or three times a day for a few days at a time, probably relieves the attack by mobilizing the individual's own adrenalin—the secretion of the adrenal glands. This recommendation applies only to Kalion (Neoco), not to commercial potassium chloride, which is difficult to dissolve; nausea and pain or cramp or irritation of stomach may occur if potassium chloride is taken undissolved, or if it is taken in less than a glassful of water. Kalion (Neoco) contains also vitamin C.

IS YOUR LIVER SLUGGISH?   From away back it has been the popular belief and common medical practice that a brisk saline cathartic is generally good for whatever ails the individual who is coming down with the cri. This idea probably arises from the quaint fancy that the liver is a wilful, obstinate organ anyway and it soldiers on the job whenever it finds an excuse to behave that way; hence we must be ever vigilant and take a good dose of salts whenever we fear or suspect the liver may be a bit sluggish. On this basis my liver must be in a deplorable condition, for I haven't taken any kind of salts or other physic in a coon's age and I never shall unless a better doctor than I am makes me do so.

However, if the portal area—the great network of veins carrying blood from the stomach and intestine to the liver really is congested, or overfilled with blood, from any cause, there will be more or less retarded flow and congestion in the veins carrying blood from the area of the mucous membrane of nose and throat into the great veins near the heart. This is one way in which overeating predisposes to chronic catarrh, so it is true that a brisk saline cathartic momentarily relieves nose and throat congestion due to such portal engorgement, and it is probably for this reason that a physic seems to do good in some cases of acute cri or of chronic catarrh. But such relief is of short duration, for it is a matter of a few hours before the water removed from the blood in the portal area by a dose of salts is restored. Far better to stop the overeating, the hasty eating, even to fast for part of a day or a whole day, or in chronic cases to correct the diet and the eating habits—these hygienic measures will give a lasting effect and at the same time promote improvement in general health. Adequate daily exercise, active enough to make you puff and breathe hard for a while, is valuable for the same purpose. Even a few seconds devoted to rolling a dozen somersaults first thing on getting out of bed every morning, and the regular practices of belly breathing last thing every night will do good where more vigorous exercise is not possible.

ATROPHIC RHINITIS Like a "cold" and "impure blood," "dry catarrh" is a term which serves only to conceal ignorance or to mislead. Other names for atrophic rhinitis are fetid coryza and ozena. Ozena is derived from a Greek word meaning "to smell," but odor does not always accompany atrophic rhinitis. When there is a fetid odor the patient usually believes it is from stomach trouble or a decayed tooth, and indeed both of these conditions may be present and mislead him, his physician and his dentist. Generally the patient perceives his odor slightly or not at all, because the sense of smell is partially or completely lost in atrophic rhinitis.

Dryness and irritation in the nostrils, absence of the normal mucous secretion, that serves to keep the membrane protected in health, and crust formation are characteristic symptoms of atrophic rhinitis. Hoarseness and a constant hacking cough, impairment of the sense of taste, and in some cases impairment of hearing accompany the condition.

First essential in treatment, whether the "dry catarrh" is associated with bad odor or not, is thorough cleansing of crusts and secretions from the nasal passages night and morning by means of spray, douche or irrigation. Any simple, well warmed alkaline solution may be used; a good one prepared at home is a solution of a tablespoonful of borax, a tablespoonful of sodium bicarbonate (saleratus, baking soda) and a tablespoonful of common salt (use rounded tablespoonfuls) in a pint of boiled water.

HOW TO SPRAY   In using a spray atomizer or irrigation (flow from fountain syringe reservoir) it is well to heed these general instructions:

(1) Always have the solution as warm as the body temperature or a little warmer.

(2) Stand or sit with head erect and direct spray or flow from nozzle straight back along floor of nasal passage.

(3) Learn to hold the throat and soft palate in the "k" position as when saying "hike" with the "k" sound long retained in throat; this closes the passage from the nasal chamber into the throat, so that the head may be thrown back and the solution reach the post-nasal spaces without getting back into the throat; then the head may be bent forward again while excess of solution drains from the nostrils. Once learned this same maneuver permits thorough irrigation of the nasal cavity even in infant or young child, by allowing the solution to enter through one nostril and drain from the opposite one. Such nasal irrigation is a valuable aid in treating various children's diseases, notably diphtheria and scarlet fever, where the child is too young to gargle.

(4) When using a nasal douche or irrigation do not attempt to draw the solution into the nasal passage, as that may force material into the Eustachian tubes leading to the ears and cause serious ear trouble. Merely allow the solution to flow through the passages, from a level not more than a few inches above the head.

(5) No matter whether the trouble is simple, hypertrophic or atrophic rhinitis, it is unwise to continue indefinitely the use of spray or other treatment. If cleansing or medication of the nasal mucous membrane seems necessary as a matter of habit or routine it is best to change from one agent to another from time to time. The advice and perhaps the treatment of the physician should be sought in reference to continuing the use of spray or irrigation longer than six months.

SIMPLE REMEDIES FOR OZENA A foul discharge coming from one side of the nose suggests the possibility of a foreign body lodged there, especially in the case of an infant or young child. In some instances it is a manifestation of nasal diphtheria. Occasionally the foreign body is animate—an insect, intestinal worm, even the developing larva of a fly (maggot). Most serious, even fatal symptoms are sometimes produced by the presence of an animate foreign body in the nose. Hence the importance of a careful medical examination with the aid of headlight, speculum and other instruments is obvious. The laity has been oversold on specialism. A competent general practitioner or family doctor can diagnose and treat all of these everyday nose and throat conditions as well as any what-have-you specialist can. After all, Mrs. Whitecollar and Mrs. Executive merely betray their cheap snobbery in running to the specialist every time the baby—well, whenever a word of medical advice is needed. That sort of thing may have impressed the neighbors in the days when bloomers were news; today it is as distinctive as lipstick.

Atrophic rhinitis, or "dry catarrh," the usual cause of ozena, calls for painstaking daily cleansing of the nasal passages. This is the best way to check or control the foul odor.

Aside from the cleansing, or following such cleansing of the affected mucous membrane, one or another of the simple remedies here suggested may be used to advantage.

First, when the nose is quite clear and as free from secretion as possible, apply some precipitated sulphur by means of an insufflator or powder blower. One application of the powdered sulphur each alternate day is sufficient, and it may be continued for several weeks. This is helpful not only in simple chronic rhinitis but also in atrophic rhinitis, with or without ozena.

Second, following the cleansing of the nasal passages apply a suitable oil to soothe and protect the mucous membranes. For this purpose it is better to avoid the mineral oil preparations, such as petrolatum or paraffin oil, so often used in nasal sprays, drops, inhalants and nebulizers. One good agent for the purpose is a solution of iodine in sesame oil—one grain of iodine to the ounce of oil. Another is common kerosene. If kerosene oil seems repugnant, a purified or nearly deodorized preparation of it may be obtained from the druggist.

Many victims of chronic "dry catarrh" have experienced much benefit from spraying once or twice daily a warm solution of a rounded teaspoonful of cane sugar in two fluid ounces of water.

COME OUT OF YOUR SAHARA   Most of our American buildings are overheated with abnormally dry air in wintertime. This is a mischievous combination. The air in a building heated to 70 degrees F. or higher when the outside temperature is below freezing is drier than the driest desert air. It is this extreme dryness indoors throughout the winter season, not the cold or the dampness outdoors, that is the chief cause of chronic rhinitis, chronic pharyngitis, chronic sinusitis and chronic bronchitis. In a building which is not air-conditioned or where a reasonable amount of water is not evaporated, the higher the temperature, the drier the atmosphere . . . and the more frequent the respiratory troubles.

Although built-in air-conditioning is the most efficient and desirable way to handle the problem, any artificially heated room or building may be made more healthful and habitable by merely keeping an open reservoir of water on radiator or stove to favor evaporation. Evaporation of a gallon or two of water daily in a small room will prove well worth the trouble for anyone with any kind of chronic nose, throat or chest trouble.

POLYP   Polyps in the nose usually indicate underlying trouble in one or more of the accessory sinuses. On this account it is necessary to do more than just snare or shrivel or remove the polyp if the object is to relieve the patient of the trouble. In every instance where one or more polyps form in the nasal cavity the condition of the nasal sinuses should be carefully investigated and the inflammation or infection which is generally present in one or more sinuses vigorously treated after the polyp has been removed.

Polyp swells in damp weather, and the patient is then most conscious of the obstruction in the nose. It is necessary to mention, however, that polyp in the nose sometimes causes obstinate "laryngeal" cough and sometimes trouble resembling asthma. Polyp is easily recognized by the physician who examines with speculum, headlamp or mirror. It is useless to attempt self-diagnosis or self-treatment in any case of constant or intermittent nasal obstruction with constant discharge, with or without "laryngeal" cough—that is, a constant cough that seems to be due to irritation in the throat —and the characteristic nasal twang or lack of nasal resonance in the voice, whether polyp is present or not.

Removal of polyp in the old-fashioned way, by means of wire snare, or by cutting the mass free with scissors, is more or less painful and disagreeable. Shrinking the polyp with electro-desiccation or electro-coagulation, to produce shrivelling of the grape-like mass, is comparatively mild and as effective if not more effective than the older method.

ANY OTHER CLIMATE Referring to sinusitis (it might as well be chronic bronchitis, chronic rhinitis or "catarrh" or even lung trouble) an Iowa reader says two doctors advised operation, one advised against operation, and the doctor who is treating him now advised him to go to Arizona. The patient, however, has a job and a family in Iowa. What to do?

The grass is always greener in other pasture. There is always better fruit to be found at a stand farther on. A filling station just over the next mountain will offer better service. Wherever you happen to live, the climate is probably better elsewhere.

I have always had a suspicion, and now I am convinced, that the only advantage of one climate over another lies in the fact that you can wear less clothing and absorb more sunshine—ultraviolet light, vitamin D—in one climate than in another.

Of course the more cloud, fog, smoke or dust in the air the less sunshine reaches the earth. This is one reason why respiratory diseases are so prevalent among the poorer city dwellers in industrial cities where the air is constantly heavily laden with smoke, carbon, acid, ash, and one reason why chronic "catarrh," chronic bronchitis, chronic sinusitis and similar troubles are difficult to cure.

Dampness or moisture makes extreme cold more penetrating and extreme heat more oppressive. Well or sick, you can stand or enjoy very hot or very cold weather better if the air is comparatively dry; you are more readily chilled when the air is heavily saturated with water vapor, enervated more quickly if the hot weather is accompanied by high humidity.

Literally tons of literature, some of it purely medical, some promotional, most of it a shrewd combination of the two, deals with the advantages of climate. Having watched people for years I have been impressed by the salutary influence of any climate far from home.

In my judgment the actual benefits invalids and valetudinarians gain with change of climate are (1) more exposure to sunlight, (2) better air-conditioning, and (3) evading or escaping an environment which may be an important factor of trouble at home.

Some of the same benefits may be had anywhere by (a) spending more time out of doors, or (b) regulating household heating by thermometer or thermostat rather than personal fancy or whim and using any adequate means to evaporate a reasonable amount of water in the artificially heated air of your building each 24 hours during the heating season.

Another benefit of change of climate may be illustrated by a specific case. A woman suffered more or less constantly from asthma while living in Hamilton, Ontario. One winter she went to Southern California and obtained great relief immediately upon arrival, had no trouble for about three months, returned home and suffered an attack the very next day. A few months later she happened to visit friends in Niagara Falls, N.Y., 40 miles east of Hamilton. Her breathing was easy and no wheezing occurred during the two weeks she remained 40 miles from home. But within 24 hours after her return home the old wheeze came back. These peculiar reactions aroused her doctor's suspicions. He investigated her domestic environment, discovered a parrot, made a skin test, obtained a characteristic reaction (hive-like swelling around the point where the homeopathic quantity of parrot feather was scratched in) and persuaded the patient's husband to dispatch the raucous bird. Within the week the asthma cleared up and has never returned. Had the lady made her home in California or in Niagara Falls, leaving the parrot behind, she might have become a living testimonial for the climate of either place where she recovered her health as contrasted with the "damp" climate of home.

Chapter Sixteen

A LOOK AT SINUSITIS, LARYNGITIS AND BRONCHITIS

In the bones of the skull there are four pair of air-spaces which communicate with the nasal passages. These are the maxillary sinuses or antra in the upper jaw bones, the frontal sinuses just above the orbits behind the brows, the ethmoid sinuses or cells in the roof of the nasal passages and the sphenoid sinus in the roof over the rear of the nasal cavity.

Except to give resonance to the voice, the purpose of these air-spaces is unknown. Of course the skull is lighter than it would be without them, but whether that makes it stronger or better in any way is not known. From all we hear about sinus trouble nowadays it might seem that the sinuses are designed only to keep doctors and specialists busy; but in fact there is no reason to imagine sinus trouble of any kind is more frequent today than it has always been. It is more commonly recognized or diagnosed today, that is all. Sinusitis is in no sense a new disease, but merely a refinement in the diagnosis of an ailment that formerly passed as "brow ague," supraorbital "neuralgia" or facial "neuralgia," "headache," or even "toothache" in many cases of maxillary sinusitis particularly.

Each of the sinuses communicates through a small opening with the nasal cavity. Since it is lined with mucous membrane continuous with the lining of the nasal cavity, the sinuses are likely to share in any nasal inflammation. If the opening from a sinus into the nasal passage becomes nearly or quite closed, as by swelling of the mucous membrane around it, the secretion in the sinus can no longer drain into the nose as it does normally. With accumulation of excessive mucus or, following infection, muco-pus or purulent fluid, pain of greater or less intensity occurs.

One or more of the sinuses become inflamed with every acute coryza, cri or "cold in the head." Such simple acute sinusitis is the usual explanation for more than ordinarily profuse muco-purulent discharge from the nose after acute coryza, or for unduly prolonged discharge of such thick secretion. Complicating frontal or antral sinusitis accounts also for the actual tenderness or pain felt in the brow or behind the cheek or between the eyes at the height of the attack of acute coryza, rhinitis or "grippe."

Antral or maxillary sinusitis is the commonest. This may come from extension of infection from the nose, or from the root of one of the upper teeth, particularly a second bicuspid or first molar, whose roots often project into the floor of the sinus and are separated from the space by only a thin wall of bone and mucous membrane. Advantage of this proximity is taken in the treatment of maxillary sinusitis by drainage or irrigation of the sinus through the socket of such a tooth, though drainage of the sinus through the nasal passage is generally more satisfactory in effect.

Injuries and inflammation of nose, eyes or teeth sometimes give rise to complicating sinusitis, but the cause of sinusitis is almost invariably an extension of inflammation or infection from the nasal mucous membrane into one or more of the sinuses.

Why acute or chronic rhinitis extends into the sinuses in some cases and not in others is a question for speculation. We shall say nothing about "lowered resistance," because that is sheer blah anyway and doctors who mention it as a predisposing factor of any disease are simply indulging in pretense. No physician can define resistance, apart from immunity, and no one can speak intelligently of immunity unless he refers specifically to the infection he has in mind—say typhoid, diphtheria, tetanus or smallpox. I mean to say there is no such condition as general immunity against disease recognized in science.

Probably the factors we have already considered as causes of chronic rhinitis are also causes of chronic sinusitis. As for diet, notwithstanding the many books and pamphlets issued by doctors, regular and irregular, it is my conviction that overeating is the important dietary factor of chronic sinusitis, and any benefit a sinusitis sufferer obtains from dieting is attributable to the reduced intake of calories the dietary restrictions entail.

Calcium shortage is far more likely to favor the development and chronic appearance of sinusitis than is any fancied "acidosis" or preponderance of acid ash. My dietary prescription for the individual subject to chronic sinusitis therefore is this:

(1) If you are past 30, reduce your daily caloric intake by cutting out, say, dessert after a square meal or sugar in tea or coffee or on fruit or one slice of bread or toast.

(2) Take not less than a quart of fresh milk a day, certified if it is available and you can afford it, Grade A Raw from tuberculin tested herd as second choice, Grade A Pasteurized if the better grades are not available to you. Of course it doesn't matter whether you drink the milk straight or take part or all of it in various dishes or combinations.

(3) Include in your diet not less than an egg a day cooked as you prefer or raw if you like, or six or eight eggs once a week if you prefer.

(4) Two raw vegetables, at least one raw fruit, and some nuts or peanuts in place of dessert daily.

As vitamin D is essential for the assimilation and utilization of calcium and phosphorus, an adequate intake of vitamin D should always accompany calcium feeding. A combination of vitamin D with calcium, ideal for supplementing the diet, is Calcicaps (Nion). Six may be taken daily for a ten weeks period in any case where calcium deficiency is to be corrected.

CONSERVATIVE TREATMENT OF SINUSITIS   In severe acute sinusitis where there are symptoms or signs of suppuration, empyema, pus formation or abscess, especially if there are associated general indications of septicemia or septic poisoning, prompt surgical relief is the most conservative treatment. But for ordinary acute sinusitis the simpler and milder the local treatment the better as a rule, except for careful application of medicinal agents by the physician to shrink the swollen mucous membrane.

Otherwise the best treatment for acute sinusitis is the same as treatment for acute cri—hot bath, bed, plenty of hot or cool drinks —soup, milk, fruit juice beverages, or a 12 to 24 hour fast if you remain in bed; the fool-proof cough medicine as described earlier; one grain of quinine for every 50 pounds of your body weight every four hours; a dose of five or ten grains of aspirin, repeated if necessary in two hours, if any pain-killer is used at all.

Among the resources of the physician who treats nose and throat diseases, ultraviolet irradiation applied by special apparatus within the nasal cavity, as well as ultrashort wave diathermy or radiothermy treatment is efficacious in many cases of chronic sinusitis. X-ray treatment is of questionable value, though x-ray negatives do aid in the precise diagnosis of sinusitis.

There are innumerable preparations—solutions, oils, sprays, vaporizers, inhalants, salves, drops—offered as remedies for chronic sinus trouble. The more effective of these generally depend on adrenalin or ephedrin for their characteristic action—shrinking swollen mucous membranes for a short time.

Experience has demonstrated that repeated or prolonged use of such powerful vasoconstrictors as adrenalin or ephedrin eventually leaves the mucous membrane in an abnormal condition, perhaps worse than before.

I'd take plenty of time to consider before I'd submit to any surgical treatment if I were subject to chronic sinusitis. The results of such operations are not encouraging. Too often the patient is scared into agreement when the nose and throat man says "Boo!," then regrets his hasty decision through years and years of constant or recurring trouble.

One nose and throat specialist who achieved his skill through wide experience in general practice informs me he has never been able to employ diathermy for the extirpation of tonsils, perhaps, as he concedes, because he has never mastered the technique of the method. On the other hand he has found diathermy (electro-coagulation, electro-desiccation, electro-surgery, endothermy) a most gratifying advancement in the treatment of sinusitis; so much preferable to the older surgical measures that it has become the method of choice in his practice.

In urging the advisability of conservative treatment I do not mean to say that surgery is never necessary or advisable, nor that diathermy is always preferable to more radical surgical operation. My purpose is merely to warn the public against certain shrewd merchants who hold themselves out to the public as "specialists."

In long standing cases of sinusitis the thyroid gland function seems to become exhausted. This calls for either the iodine ration or, if the patient's temperature is below the normal 98 between 4 and 6 P.M. daily, small daily doses of thyroid extract—the thyroid extract should be discontinued if or when the body weight shows a loss or the pulse rate, which has been slow, is more than 90 a minute when the patient is at rest. Of course, thyroid extract can be safely used only under the observation of the physician.

The general hygiene, diet, clothing, ventilation, sunshine, air-conditioning, heating, constitutional remedies advisable for sufferers from chronic sinusitis are the same as those advisable for sufferers from other chronic respiratory diseases such as chronic bronchitis, and we'll consider them in the section on bronchitis.

Regular or systematic use of sprays, douches, irrigations or suction is as likely to harm as it is to help. Such treatment should be restricted to occasions or periods when the physician specifically prescribes it.

TRACHEITIS IS LARYNGITIS, BRONCHITIS IS AS BAD   The medical name for the windpipe is trachea. The upper part of the trachea is the voice-box or larynx. The prominence of the cartilage forming the larynx is commonly known as the Adam's apple. At this lower end the windpipe divides into the bronchi, two tubes leading to the right and left lungs.

Inflammation of the windpipe lining is called tracheitis; inflammation of the voice box lining is called laryngitis; inflammation of the tubes into which the trachea divides is bronchitis, whether the inflammation is confined to the two main tubes or extends into their smaller divisions going to all parts of the lungs.

Characteristic of acute laryngitis is hoarseness or temporary loss of voice, with much unproductive coughing in the early stage.

Essential treatment is (a) absolute rest of voice, which means not even the attempt to whisper—this silence is what makes acute laryngitis so dreadful for certain people; (b) cold moist compresses on the Adam's apple; (c) Old Doctor Brady's Foolproof Cough Medicine every two hours; (d) every hour or two, inhalation for a few minutes of the steam or vapor arising from a pitcher or old coffee pot of boiling water into which a tablespoonful of compound tincture of benzoin has been stirred.

All of these measures are equally helpful in acute tracheitis or acute bronchitis. In any such acute illness, especially if accompanied with chilliness or chills and fever, a hot mustard bath administered to the patient in bed by a nurse or other trained person, is always beneficial in the early stage. Next best general measure of alleviation is a hot bath before the patient gets into bed. The purpose of either is simply to equalize the circulation, withdraw blood to the surface from the congested areas.

A remedial factor of importance commonly overlooked is air-conditioning. Whatever means will increase the amount of water vapor in the air will add materially to the patient's comfort. Excessively dried out, artificially heated air is irritating to the inflamed mucous membrane of larynx, trachea or bronchial tubes.

It is a serious, sometimes a fatal mistake to resort to any narcotic, nerve sedative or sense-benumbing drug in the early stage of any acute respiratory disease. The irritation and cough should be relieved rather by the measures suggested above.

In my judgment there is no advantage in taking saline or other cathartics or laxatives in the early stage of such illness, except in the presence of unusual complications.

From scientific study and from long observation I am convinced that it doesn't matter whether the patient takes milk, soups, weak tea or coffee, lemonade or other fruit juice beverages hot or cold. As long as plenty of fluid is taken the patient's individual preference should decide whether it shall be hot or cold.

BRONCHIAL TROUBLE   Chronic bronchitis, the familiar winter cough of the aged, follows repeated attacks of acute bronchitis or develops gradually in persons who are subject to heart disease, kidney disease or chronic lung trouble. In any case when acute bronchitis keeps a patient ill more than two weeks, it is well to have a careful examination made to see what the first diagnosis has missed.

The ancients, from Hippocrates to Dr. Osler, believed that the regularly recurring winter cough of chronic bronchitis was due to the cold and changeable weather. Plenty of doctors today harbor quaint ideas about it. But we can't accept a theory as sound just because it is old. The medical profession ought to be first to acknowledge this. It seems more sensible to believe that if you are subject to chronic bronchial trouble—bronchitis, bronchiectasis (dilation or ballooning of bronchial tubes), bronchial asthma or emphysema (ballooning of the air-cells of the lungs from loss of elasticity or resiliency)—you will feel worse during the season of artificial heating because (a) the indoor atmosphere is so excessively dried out and (b) you get so little sunshine vitamin D all winter. Anyway this concept has some logic in it, whereas the old concept had none at all that could satisfy a rational mind. Well knowing that most physicians or health authorities still share the view of Hippocrates and Osler, I give you my earnest conviction that dampness, wet feet, sudden change of weather, drafts and cold neither cause acute respiratory diseases nor predispose to them.

Dusts produced by nature and by numerous industries are a factor of all acute respiratory diseases. The respiratory disease caused in various occupations by coal dust, stone dust and iron dust is well known. Textile dusts are less injurious but often cause asthma, as do the dust of feathers, fur, hair or dander in persons who happen to be hypersensitive. Pollen dust of course causes hay fever as well as asthma. Air-conditioning greatly improves the air in respect to the dust hazard within buildings, but no mask or other device to protect against dust or pollen out of doors is practical or comfortable for regular use.

Perhaps the best protection against the dust you inhale day by day is the normal secretion of mucus by the lining of the breathing passages. This mucus not only guards against germs invading the mucous membrane, but also entangles grains of dust or pollen and eventually extrudes them from the body, either by way of the alimentary tract or by direct discharge from the nose. This is the reason why I advise against the use of sprays, douches or irrigations of the nasal passages as a means of preventing respiratory infection. I believe the normal mucous secretion is far more efficient than any such "internal bathing" for prophylaxis.

A WORD OR TWO ABOUT DISEASES MANIFEST BY COUGHS AND WHEEZES   If you are subject to chronic bronchitis, bronchiectasis or emphysema you should never forget that a certain amount of coughing is beneficial for two reasons: first, it improves circulation in abdomen and thorax; second, it is a necessary aid to expectoration or drainage from the breathing passages. It is a serious error therefore to take or do anything to check coughs unless under the immediate care of the physician.

In some cases of chronic winter cough attended with wheezing, small daily doses of iodide or iodine somewhat larger than the dose in the iodine ration are helpful. In all cases of chronic bronchitis, bronchiectasis or emphysema as well as bronchial or spasmodic asthma, the patient should in my judgment have a regular iodine ration. The attending physician should prescribe the iodide or iodine if more than the amount in the iodine ration is to be taken.

The real trouble in some cases purporting to be chronic bronchitis or recurring winter cough is neglected chronic sinusitis. Some astonishing cures are obtained by the discovery of underlying sinus infection and its drainage.

Two or three drops of purified oil of turpentine (not the crude spirits of turpentine intended for industrial use), on a little sugar or in capsule, taken twice daily after food, is an old and useful remedy in many cases of chronic cough. The turpentine derivative called terpin hydrate is perhaps easier to take—I do not know whether it is as efficient medicinally—and may be substituted in doses of two or three grains in capsule or tablet, after food, for six weeks twice a year.

The Belly Breathing exercise three or four times a day is helpful in all chronic chest diseases manifested by cough and wheeze.

In any chronic cough with expectoration the patient should assume an inverted position for five minutes every morning. Lie prone across bed with your forearms resting on the floor. This is especially helpful in bronchiectasis and emphysema.

Any means of maintaining a fair degree of humidity in the air, by evaporating water, especially during the season when artificial heating is necessary, tends to soothe or rather to prevent undue irritation of the breathing passages and should be used for victims of chronic cough or wheeze.

CROUP   Ordinary croup, sometimes called spasmodic, sometimes catarrhal croup, is a spasm of muscles in the throat induced by the irritation of a comparatively trifling coryza, sore throat or laryngitis in a child. In children such local muscle spasm, or general muscle spasms, convulsions, are more likely to occur from causes which in adults would produce only chilliness or perhaps nervous restlessness, for the nervous system of the child weighs much more in proportion to body weight.

Simple croup is alarming, but NEVER fatal. If the spasm is so severe as to imperil breathing, the inevitable result is faintness or stupor which relaxes the spasm and brings relief. Parents should bear in mind that croup never kills.

Many years ago cases of diphtheria affecting the larynx were sometimes mistaken for croup and proper treatment therefore not given. Of course this laryngeal diphtheria is likely to prove fatal unless promptly diagnosed and treated with huge doses of antitoxin. It was wrongly called "false croup" or "membranous croup"—but to use such titles today implies inexcusable ignorance.

In simple croup the child has a slight cough or running nose and perhaps becomes irritable or a little feverish toward bedtime. After a night or two the crowing breathing of the attack comes on. The attack passes and the child is not ill next day, though the croup is likely to recur for two or three nights. This is very different from diphtheria or "membranous croup" for in this disease the child grows increasingly ill from the first and is no better next morning —the difficulty of breathing is not limited to several minutes, as it usually is in true croup, but is persistent and unrelenting for hours and days and nights on end.

I am sure no parent need feel any anxiety over croup if these marked differences between it and laryngeal diphtheria are borne in mind.

Children with adenoids or diseased tonsils are more likely to have croup than others. For such children I suggest daily rations of calcium and vitamin D—NOT removal of tonsils, at least not just for croup.

Children who sleep in cold rooms, with window and door wide open, are practically immune to croup. I have never seen croup occur in a properly ventilated sleeping apartment. Of course, the child must be warmly covered.

The best remedy I know for croup, if the night happens to be a cool or cold one, is to wrap the child in a blanket and sit with him for a while by the window or on a porch. Understand, I do not advise exposing the child to cold. Keep the child comfortably covered and permit it to have the sedative, relaxing, quieting effect of pure cold night air.

Another excellent remedy is the constant application of compresses moistened with ice water to the front of the neck over the larynx (the Adam's apple region). These should be changed every two minutes and continued for half an hour or longer.

Syrup of ipecac is the time-honored croup remedy, a teaspoonful being the usual emetic dose for a young child. The vomiting usually does not occur for ten or fifteen minutes after the dose is given, but the act of vomiting, however produced, necessarily relaxes the throat muscles and so relieves the attack.

As soon as a child develops any symptoms of croup begin giving it Fool Proof Cough Medicine every two hours.

Tetany, spasmophilia, enlarged tonsils and adenoids are frequent states in children subject to attacks of croup. For prevention and correction of any and all of these states as well as the tendency to croup, I advise that every growing child should be given a suitable daily ration of calcium and vitamin D to supplement the regular diet which is nearly always deficient in these nutritional essentials. For instance, let the child eat a Calciwafer (Nion) once or twice daily with food the year around.

A simple, effective way to insure good ventilation in a child's sleeping-room, play-room or school-room in any weather in any climate, is by installing a full-sash window screen or screens of unbleached muslin in place of windows or in such fashion as to permit keeping a window wide open all the time. This admits light, fresh air and desirable moisture, while excluding wind, extreme cold, rain, snow, dust and insects.

Chapter Seventeen

THE TONSIL QUESTION

The four tonsils are composed of adenoid, round-cell or lymphoid tissue, the same tissue as that of the lymph nodes or "lymph glands" in various parts of the body—those nodes which, when enlarged or inflamed, are called "kernels."

The function of lymphoid tissue wherever it is found is to maintain immunity against infection. This is the consensus of physiologists and physicians.

The two faucal tonsils, one on each side of the throat, are familiar to everybody. The pharyngeal tonsil, called "adenoids" when enlarged, is located on the roof and rear wall of the naso-pharynx or post-nasal space, out of direct sight behind the soft palate. The fourth tonsil is merely a small amount of lymphoid tissue on the base or root of the tongue. Thus the airway to larynx, trachea, bronchi and lungs is ringed by lymphoid tissue which supplies what is known as round cells to the mucus secreted by the membrane lining of nose and throat. These cells act as phagocytes; that is, they eat or destroy germs and so keep the body immune from *respiratory infection*.

This, at least, is the theory—the only logical way, I believe, to account for the existence of these particular lymphoid structures in strategic areas. There is, for instance, a similar ring of lymphoid tissue in the wall of the cecum around the orifice of the vermiform appendix, and it is probably not a coincidence that acute appendicitis is a frequent complication or sequel of tonsillitis.

165

The craze for removing tonsils reached a peak in the '20s. There have been many such crazes. At one time there was a rash of appendectomies—although we must frankly acknowledge that the vermiform appendix has no known function and as far as can be determined there are no ill effects from its removal.

Then there is the gall bladder. It does have a function—to contain the bile, or gall, more or less constantly secreted by the liver until it is needed in digestion. Then the gall bladder squirts out its contents—about an ounce—into the duodenum exactly as a rubber bulb would squirt liquid. This function, however, is not very important and again many people appear to suffer no ill effects from cholecystectomy, the removal of the gall bladder.

For a while, women were having hysterectomies right and left. Recently the fashion has been for spinal fusions. In the early decades of the twentieth century some physicians and surgeons, obsessed with the "autointoxication" or "intestinal toxemia" theory, advocated and practiced surgical removal of part of the colon. They made themselves and their clients believe mankind would be better off without colons which, they claimed, served only as factories for producing all kinds of germs, poisons, toxins to pour into the blood stream and give people all kinds of evil symptoms —symptoms which might instead have been ascribed to introspection, since they came from constantly watching one's bowels. It was all pretty radical and pretty profitable, and some physicians around the world received a lot of free advertising in American magazines and Sunday supplements for changing colons into semicolons.

But to get back to the tonsil question:

When something goes wrong in that department, the operation generally preferred since the 20's has been tonsillectomy, a radical procedure which, the doctors insisted, was the only way to "get every bit of tonsil." In view of the immunological or protective functions of adenoid, round-cell or lymphoid tissue in the body I can't see why anyone should attempt to "get every bit of tonsil." For that matter, in most tonsillectomies there is more or less tonsil tissue left even after extensive dissection of the neck.

For enlarged, hypertrophied tonsils the only purpose of operating is to remove that portion of tonsil which obstructs breathing, prevents ventilation or drainage of the middle ear, deadens the voice or interferes with speech or swallowing. This is accomplished with a minimum of danger by tonsillotomy.

Tonsillotomy is instantaneous and requires a minimum of anesthesia—it is as quickly over and as easy on the patient as extraction of a tooth. It is a minor operation. Tonsillectomy on the other hand—the attempt to cut out every bit of tonsil tissue—is a major operation with numerous hazards which, in my opinion, make it unjustifiable.

In horse and buggy days, before the eager operators conceived the idea of "getting every bit of tonsil," simple tonsillotomy, often done in the doctor's office, was the standard, uniformly satisfactory way of treating enlarged tonsils. We never heard of such dreadful complications as fatal hemorrhage, cardiac arrest (cessation of heart beat), lodgment of a piece of tonsil or throat tissue in bronchus or lung, collapse of lung (atelectasis), pneumonia, or lung abscess. I wouldn't mention such hazards if tonsillectomies were necessary. Indeed, I would rather tell a lie than frighten parents about necessary surgery. But in this instance I hope every parent who reads this diatribe will be sufficiently frightened never to consent to perpetration of this atrocity on a child.

On November 28, 1959 no less than ten doctors signed a letter to the editor of the New Haven Journal-Courier, published in the Readers' forum, characterizing one of my articles about tonsillectomy as "vicious." It was vicious, they said, because "it creates in people, especially parents of children who need tonsillectomy" (the doctors really said "tonsillectomies"—the more the merrier), "such an uncalled for horror of the contemplated operation as to affect their own health adversely in unnecessary worry."

That was precisely my purpose. It still is. The New England doctors seemed especially upset by my statement that tonsillectomy has a "frightfully high death rate" which, they said, is completely wrong.

I don't know how high the death rate would have to be for these courageous defenders of tonsil-snatching to consider it frightful. It frightens me just to look at a handful of newspaper reports of tonsillectomy fatalities. "Patrolman's three and a half year old son who died early yesterday in a local hospital after a tonsillec-

tomy . . ." "Three-year-old daughter of _____ died suddenly in _____ General Hospital following a tonsil and adenoid
operation." "Beauty queen of _____ High School died five
hours after operation to remove her tonsils." "Boy, 12, died un-
expectedly following tonsil operation." "Six-year-old son of ____
_____ died Friday night when his heart stopped, following a
routine tonsillectomy." "Six-year-old _____ died in
hospital here 15 hours after he underwent tonsillectomy, and three
other children, aged four years, two years and ten months respec-
tively, died following tonsillectomy in the same area recently."
"Miss _____, 21, died while having her tonsils removed
under anesthesia; the medical examiner found the cause of death
'difficult to determine'." "Patrolman _____, aged 28, died
during removal of tonsils; doctors said cardiac arrest caused death."
In other words the patrolman's heart stopped beating. "Inspector
_____ of the police automobile detail died suddenly after
tonsillectomy; heart failure was given as the cause of death." "Five-
year-old boy who, with his two and a half-year-old brother, underwent tonsillectomy, died four hours after the operation without
regaining consciousness." "College swimmer died on the operating
table during tonsillectomy; he had entered the hospital for 'what
is usually considered a minor operation.' "

Anyone who considers tonsillectomy a minor operation should
have his head examined. That is just a conventional lie which
knife-happy operators tell parents when persuading them to sacrifice children to the bloody Moloch.

Now I repeat that tonsillectomy is *not* a minor operation. It is
a *major operation,* with all the hazards of major surgery. The
fatalities enumerated above are taken at random from a fat file
of newspaper reports, but even if they comprised the total mortality
figures for tonsillectomy I would call the death rate frightfully high.

A New Jersey mother writes:

"I took my daughter, not quite five, to the hospital to have her
tonsils removed because she had so much trouble with colds and
sore throat. She was in perfect health . . ."

(Please pardon the interruption, but if the child was in perfect health why subject her to major surgery?) But to go back to the letter:

"No one told me the operation was dangerous and I never heard of a child dying of it. That is, not until I was called by the hospital early next morning and told that she was dead. They could not explain _____ said everyone that had been in the operating-room at the time had been shaken. . . .

I wish that you had written your article about tonsillectomy a month ago. It might have saved. . . ."

(Signed) Mrs. _____

The trouble is, Ma'am, that if you had read the article a month ago it would probably have made little impression on your mind, or perhaps you would have smiled and thought how opinionated this old doctor was.

In reference to tonsils I must confess I am opinionated. But then, the significance and treatment of enlarged or infected tonsils is necessarily a matter of the doctor's opinion.

Examining the throat a year after tonsillectomy physicians find in most cases more or less tonsil intact. This is of no consequence except that it makes the claim of "getting every bit of tonsil" ridiculous.

No one had warned this unhappy mother that tonsillectomy was dangerous. Yet it invariably involves the hazards or dangers I have already mentioned, so that no physician, surgeon or specialist can honestly assure parents that even in skilled hands tonsillectomy is entirely free from risk or danger. For we just can't write off the surgeons, anesthetists and other assistants in the fatal cases mentioned as unskilled.

Whether or not a patient survives tonsillectomy is beside the point. The point I am making is this: In my opinion there is no good reason why a patient should be subjected to tonsillectomy at all, when instantaneous tonsillotomy serves every purpose the most pretentious tonsillectomy does, with no greater risk than might be involved in extraction of a tooth.

The New Jersey mother had been made to believe removal of the child's tonsils would prevent recurring "colds" and sore throat. This same fond hope has made thousands of parents consent to have children tonsillectomized. But the best statistics we have, the observations of Dr. Albert D. Kaiser (*Children's Tonsils In and Out,* J. B. Lippincott Company—the book should be available in your library) indicate that removal of tonsils and adenoids makes little if any difference in the frequency of "colds" and sore throat in school children. Most healthy school children have two or three such illnesses in the course of the school year, whether they have had tonsil operations or not. So the doctor who promises or implies that tonsillectomy, or for that matter just tonsillotomy, will put an end to the child's repeated "colds" is merely exploiting popular credulity.

Over a period of many years I have had scores of pieces in my column deploring the perpetration of tonsillectomy on children. From the outburst of the ten New England doctors who called my teaching vicious I gather that *some* parents have enough confidence in me to hold back a bit when the ever-ready operator wants to operate immediately. But the majority of parents who happen to notice what I say about tonsillectomy are not at the moment confronted with the problem so they scarcely know what we're talking about. That's the way my ten New England colleagues like 'em.

Seldom if ever do adenoids occur without enlargement of the faucal tonsils. Moreover, the morbid effects or symptoms produced by adenoids are indistinguishable from those produced by enlargement of the tonsils. Also it is routine practice when doing a tonsillotomy to scrape or curette any adenoid "vegetations" which may be present. The name "vegetations" is a misnomer, for the lymphoid tissue which composes tonsils or adenoids is not a new growth, but merely overgrowth or enlargement of the normal lymphatic structures.

Some of the symptoms or effects produced by enlarged tonsils and/or adenoids are mouth breathing, particularly at night, difficulty in swallowing, perhaps regurgitation of foods and liquids, more or less deafness which makes the child seem stupid, restless nights, night-terrors, expressionless face, nasal twang, faulty pronunciation of consonants which may lead to stuttering, rasping, hacking cough at night, and tendency toward croup or asthma.

Addison, N.Y., is a village of perhaps 3000 population. Lucky are the kids who grow up there or in any other village that size, rather than in a large city. In the '20s, when I lived in Buffalo, Dr. Wm. E. Barron of Addison, in his capacity as health officer or maybe school physician, examined all the pupils in one school, late in the spring, and found many of them had enlarged tonsils. The doctor advised their parents to seek medical treatment.

After the summer vacation the doctor again examined the same pupils. Few if any of them had received medical attention but nearly all now had normal tonsils. Reporting this experience in the *N. Y. State Journal of Medicine* (I didn't know Dr. Barron and he didn't know me, so the editor of the Journal permitted publication of his report), Dr. Barron expressed his astonishment. I was astonished, too. And ever since then I have counseled parents to take it easy when some one wants to remove those "bad" tonsils. Give the youngster a break—a summer with a minimum of clothing, for instance. This generally takes care of enlarged tonsils just a little bit better than the surgeon can. If the youngster spends the summer as nearly naked as the neighbors will permit his tonsils will probably be okay by Labor Day.

What might be called conservative treatment of enlarged tonsils, by repeated applications of iodine, acids, electrocautery or diathermy is generally not satisfactory.

Diathermy (electro-coagulation or electro-desiccation), however, is in my judgment the method of choice for the treatment of *infected* tonsils. The purpose of treatment here is merely to pasteurize, disinfect, destroy or drain the infected area. It is wrong to imagine and it would be atrocious to attempt to *remove* tonsils by diathermy.

If lymphoid tissue in the tonsils or elsewhere in the body serves any other purpose than to defend against infection, physiologists have not determined what it may be. Because we know lymphoid tissue guards the body from invasion by disease germs, I maintain it is fortunate for the victim of tonsillectomy that the operator usually does NOT "get every bit of tonsil." If a fair portion or portions of tonsil are left in the throat after the atrocity, the result will be nearly as good as it is after tonsillotomy, which leaves most of the tonsil intact.

Examination of 1000 tonsils removed by fairly good physicians and specialists showed that many of the tonsils removed were normal and free from infection, and in some instances pieces of throat muscle were inadvertently removed along with the tonsils. It would seem that tonsils are not always as bad as they are reputed to be.

The day of Saturday morning tonsil parties is past, I hope— busloads or truckloads of hapless children corralled by teachers, social service workers and sometimes even nurses, and taken to a "clinic" for mass tonsillectomy. One Saturday morning by some odd chance an honest doctor served as substitute for a regular assembly line worker. The young patients were wheeled into the operating-room already under anesthesia—tonsil snatchers are fast workers. Suddenly the doctor startled the small audience attending the "clinic" that morning by demanding to know what one particular boy was doing there—his throat and tonsils were perfectly normal. No one could account for the youngster's presence unless perhaps he had just come along for the ride! Yet it seemed more likely that the boy's rather dull expression had misled the social worker who had decided he needed surgery.

For it was common practice, while the tonsillectomy craze was raging, for second rate doctors, nurses, school teachers and social service workers to diagnose adenoids merely by observing the child's facial expression. Textbooks of the era described the "adenoid facies"—open mouth, receding chin, dull eyes, shortened upper lip, listless expression and narrow nostrils. Although the "adenoid facies" was associated with enlargement of the third or pharyngeal tonsil, it was in fact just as likely to indicate obstruction of the breathing by other causes.

According to hackneyed newspaper stories illustrated with what purport to be humorous pictures of the victims, wholesale tonsillectomy is still perpetrated on offspring of ill-informed or uninformed people, on the group insurance or cheaper-by-the-dozen plan. Sometimes the quack who "officiates" at such performances is content with mention of his name in the story, which of course is better advertising than money can buy, and sometimes he even manages to get his picture in the paper, complete with stethoscope or head-mirror. He figures, perhaps correctly, that this will bring him enough business to compensate for the loss of professional standing or prestige such behavior entails.

Away back when I was a medical student the General Hospital, a block from the medical school, built a new surgical amphitheater lined with white tile throughout. Even the tiers of benches encircling the arena were so constructed that the entire amphitheater could be hosed out to keep it clean. They had rounded edges and corners and were shallow. It was a common occurrence for students, doctors or lay visitors sitting in the upper tiers to go limp when the operation was exceptionally, shall we say, impressive, and to come sliding downward, to be picked up and carried out.

I believe the greatest number of casualties occurred the day Dr. Roswell Park, professor of surgery and author of a two-volume *Treatise on Surgery,* operated on a four-year-old child for bow legs. The child didn't lose a drop of blood. Instead of sawing a wedge-shape section out of the main leg bone, the tibia, to permit straightening, the surgeon decided to take the anesthetized child's leg in his two hands and bend, bend, bend until the bone snapped. In the hushed amphitheater the snap was all too audible. It was followed by a chorus of groans, and a dozen spectators bit the dust.

Although I have never fainted under such circumstances I do become sick at the thought of a child being subjected to tonsillectomy. I even feel sorry for adults who submit to tonsillectomy, but I don't let that disturb me too much. After all, I have done my best these many years to warn them about it. If they do not choose to heed my warning I can only regret that I'm not as good a teacher as I ought to be. But in the entire gamut of surgery and obstetrics there is nothing so sickening to me as the plight of a child undergoing tonsillectomy. It makes me wonder whether I shouldn't have chosen some career other than medicine.

Dr. Dean J. Smiley of Cornell University found that young men who had had operations on the nose and throat were more susceptible to respiratory infections ("colds" to people who will not call them cri) than those who had not had such operations.

Dr. Warren E. Forsythe found more respiratory infections in the course of a year in tonsillectomized students than in nontonsillectomized students of the same age.

Dr. Albert D. Kaiser states in his book *Children's Tonsils In and Out* that the most common complaint of childhood is the so-called head cold. From 40 to 60 percent of preschool children have three or more "colds" a year. "Colds become less frequent from six to ten years and still less at the high school age. This natural decline in the incidence of "colds" must be remembered when the effect of removal of tonsils and adenoids is considered. The removal of tonsils and adenoids is not a generally approved method of treating children who have repeated "colds."

Susceptibility to sore throat is something else again. Numerous authorities who have studied the question over a period of years have found that 35 to 40 percent of school children with tonsils intact do have repeated attacks of sore throat. But after removal of tonsils only three to ten percent have sore throat frequently. In other words the non-tonsillectomized children continue to have tonsillitis or sore throat ten times as frequently. From these statistics it is fair to conclude that removal of the tonsils does greatly reduce a child's susceptibility to acute sore throat and tonsillitis. In computed percentages, operation offers relief to 75 percent of children subject to repeated attacks of tonsillitis and/or sore throat, whereas less than 15 percent of children not operated on become less liable to attacks over the same period of time.

But please remember, none of the statistics cited favors tonsillectomy over tonsillotomy. Removal of more (tonsillectomy) or less (tonsillotomy) tissue is in most instances for the self-same purpose—to relieve obstruction of breathing passages from enlargement, overgrowth or hypertrophy.

Sometimes the purpose of treatment is also to pasteurize, sterilize, disinfect, drain or eradicate *infection* in the tonsil tissue. This may relieve a growing child of repeated attacks of acute sore throat, tonsillitis or quinsy and an adult of some systemic manifestation of focal infection such as recurring joint trouble apparently due to septic focus in the tonsil. In regard to the theory of focal infection I must say frankly that it is all largely speculation or conjecture, yet every little while the gains made by the patient so treated seem too spectacular to be ascribed to our ubiquitous friend, A. J. Coincidence.

Although I'm a skeptic in regard to the remedial or curative value of medicines and treatments in general, I believe tonsil-

lotomy, and even tonsillectomy if the victim survives it, is of incalculable value in the prevention of rheumatic fever (inflammatory rheumatism, acute infectious arthritis), and its serious
complication, endocarditis or valvular damage, that follows in so
many cases.

In the treatment of rheumatic fever, rheumatism, arthritis, neuritis, neuralgia, headache, migraine, so-called "cold", influenza,
"grippe", tonsillitis, acute sore throat, fever, laryngitis, sinusitis,
acute ear ache, backache, toothache, sciatica or other acute illness
attended with ache or pain, aspirin (acetyl-salicylic acid) is in
my opinion the least harmful, least dangerous analgesic (pain-
killer) we have; that is, aspirin taken straight or mixed with other
pain-killers or alkalis (antacids) or sedatives or tranquilizers, as
in various popular and prescription nostrums. But I warn you,
don't let your favorite TV or radio announcer, or the headlamp or
stethoscope wearing salesman in the barber coat, tell you that this
or that kind of aspirin or aspirin mixture has any remedial value
other than temporary relief of ache or pain. From time to time some
Smart Alice, hypnotized by her pediatrician, writes to enlighten
me about this. The moment her hapless child shows a rise in temperature she begins giving it small doses of aspirin, with the blessing of her specialist. This invariably breaks the fever before it can
become established—or something to that effect. Alice usually
suggests that a post-graduate course might modernize my thinking.

From what readers tell me I gather that many doctors have
simplified the treatment of acute sore throat or tonsillitis without
loss of revenue: They give the patient an injection of penicillin
immediately, and nothing much else. This, readers seem to think,
clears up the sore throat or tonsillitis in a few days; but in a month
or so little Johnny has another sore throat and another injection
of penicillin, which is pretty expensive, and there seems to be no
end to it.

Except for the penicillin, which may tend to oppose natural im-
munization, the story is familiar—three or four attacks of sore
throat or tonsillitis in the course of the winter. Before penicillin
these illnesses cleared up in a few days on their own. I do not say
penicillin is not a good remedy. I merely say I think it has been

greatly overrated. For that matter nearly all the "wonder drugs" have been grossly overexploited and it is a wonder why doctors continue to prescribe these outrageously expensive nostrums even after they have proved worthless or dangerous.

Chapter Eighteen

THE ASPIRIN EATERS

In the halcyon days when Tony was a pup, early one November we drove from Buffalo to Beverly Hills. We drove through two days of steady rain. As luck would have it, the windshield wiper failed to work and I had to work it by hand. I suppose we might have stopped somewhere and had the thing repaired, but in the rain we didn't see a place to stop. By the time we arrived in Beverly Hills I had right sub-acromial bursitis—inflammation of the bursa or sac under the point of the shoulder.

Ow-wow, ow-wow! I learned several things from that bursitis. First, I learned to have more sympathy—if you can imagine me feeling sympathy—for other poor ginks who have it. I had always wondered why bursitis cases made such a to-do over their piddling little lameness and I had conceived a notion that perhaps they were just naturally cantankerous and their predilection for bursitis was coincidental.

Well, sir, you will be pleased to know that I got my come-uppance. The first few days in Beverly Hills I bore up admirably. But the third or fourth night a fuss became imperative. When you can no longer do your daily rolls it's high time to consult a physician. This had not occurred to me yet, but I cried so piteously at night that my family decided to do something about it. They called in a doctor who lived near by. It took him all of 30 seconds to decide we were not trying to entrap him. Then he gave me about half a barrel of something—I suppose it was morphine—and I had a fine, restful night.

The doctor repeated the dose the next night and maybe even a third, I can't remember. Then he advised me that when the pain occurred again I should eat aspirin, eat enough of it to keep me fairly comfortable.

I followed his advice, but found that ten grains three times a day and perhaps once or twice in the night did keep me quite comfortable. I had never quite realized before just how good an analgesic aspirin is.

In a week or so I needed no more aspirin—there was no more pain, just lameness and stiffness. It took several months of treatment, chiefly applications of diathermy to the shoulder followed by passive movements (manipulation of the arm by a physical therapist, to the limit of tolerance each day) and later active movements (voluntary exercise) to restore the shoulder to normal, with full range of movement.

A year later when I sustained a fracture of the left shoulder and X-ray pictures of both shoulders were made for comparison, I found that the right subacromial bursa was calcified. It may be yet, for all I know or care—the shoulder function has been normal ever since the bursitis. I mention this in case you are concerned about calcification or calcium "deposits" in or around a joint.

Prior to my discovery that aspirin would relieve bursitis pain, I had regarded it as useful only for the pain of headache and neuralgia. I do recollect I was once impressed by the experience of a young patient who had a carbuncle on the back of his neck. The medicines I prescribed gave him little or no relief. On his own he resorted to aspirin and got grateful relief for the first time in several days and nights. I don't know why I didn't learn my lesson then—I suppose I was stubborn and dismissed it as coincidence.

It is especially notable that press bulletins issued by the *Arthritis and Rheumatism Foundation* iterate and reiterate that aspirin is virtually the only medicine that will give a person with chronic joint disability (call it what you will) any satisfaction. As for the raft of newfangled, outrageously expensive nostrums the merchants of medicine prescribe for their credulous "arthritis" customers, the

Foundation says: "The various drugs in use today have not shown conclusively that they can alter the natural couse of the disease" (arthritis) "or prevent crippling." True. But what the "wonder drugs" can do is convert your bank account to small change and give your trick specialist another symbol of success.

Some 60 or 70 years ago aspirin was a proprietary or trademark name for acetyl-salicylic acid, but today anybody may make and sell aspirin and various manufacturers do. Aspirin is aspirin, no matter who makes or sells it, so when I buy aspirin I choose the cheapest kind I can find.

Although aspirin is the least dangerous analgesic or pain-killer we have, it is nevertheless poisonous to some persons. In fact as little as five or ten grains of aspirin has caused the death of a child, yet an adult who swallowed 100 five-grain tablets, apparently with suicidal intent, suffered no serious consequences.

In some instances aspirin, even in small doses, produces nausea, heartburn, feelings of weakness, collapses or angioneurotic swellings (giant hives) of face or throat or skin rashes.

There's little sense in eating aspirin or feeding it to anyone as a remedy or cure for just any ailment. It relieves unbearable ache or pain and that's all. You can't feed aspirin to your children for "cold", sore throat, fever or whatnot "with your doctor's blessing" —not if he knows therapeutics. It may well be that the indiscriminate use of aspirin as a remedy for fever, "cold" or sore throat has been promoted by a familiar trick of the trade. Doctors who want to retire to a life of leisure at 50 hate to desert good cash customers in the office and go out to make a home call for a fraction of the fees the cash customers would have paid. So they stand off the call by instructing mother to give the patient aspirin and they'll try to get around to making a visit later.

To the best of my recollection I have never taken a dose of aspirin except that once when I had bursitis. If I ever do take another I'll be cautious about it, as I think every one who takes aspirin or any other analgesic should be. By cautious I mean you should take it only when you can remain lying down or sitting quietly at rest for at least half an hour, even better full hour, afterward.

To me the habit of taking aspirin for any and every ache, pain or discomfort denotes a weak, unstable character, but as drug habits go it is not very serious. The trouble is that the aspirin eater is likely sooner or later to switch to some other drug such as acetanilid or one of the dozens of nostrums in which acetanilid is the chief ingredient. This can create real danger. The aspirin habit as such is only bad because in the first place it undermines gumption and in the second encourages you to evade medical examination, which may be necessary to determine and correct whatever makes you eat aspirin in the first place. I am bound to admit, however, that in most instances there is little or no evidence of chronic poisoning by aspirin.

Chronic acetanilid poisoning, on the other hand, is becoming a serious everyday malady, although the medical profession, the hospitals, the business interests and the press maintain a conspiracy of silence to keep the public uninformed about it.

Acetanilid destroys red blood corpuscles and interferes with the vital oxygen-carrying function of the hemoglobin, the iron coloring matter in the red corpuscles. This accounts for the cyanosis—blueness or purple color of skin, lips, nails—characteristic of acetanilid poisoning. A typical case of chronic, acute and fatal acetanilid poisoning was that of one of my bowling cronies, which I shall describe presently.

Acetanilid is the main ingredient of neuralgia and headache nostrums and of numerous so-called "cold" or "grippe" tablets. Whatever ails you, acetanilid will make you temporarily less aware of it, and if you are a blithering numskull you'll think the dope cures whatever ails you.

My friend—I might even say my benefactor, since it was he who introduced me to lawn bowling—was around 60 when he retired. He had been quite successful in business and could afford to sell out and move to this California paradise.

One of his chief interests had been a drugstore. He knew that I was a physician and had practiced for 18 years before I discovered a way to live without working and moved to paradise to do so. But the retired druggist knew me only as a playmate on the bowling green. Probably he dismissed the claim that I had practiced medicine in New York as malarkey. Anyway, he disregarded it whenever he'd explain health or medical matters to me. For instance, he told me in detail why he ate only the yolk of egg—you see, the white is albumen and Doc Somebody back East had found albumen in his urine and warned him about it. I never had the courage to tell my bowling crony that there's no more relation between eggs and kidney disease than there is between carrots and jaundice.

I never tried to tell him about the acetanilid habit either. He had acquired it when he was in the drug business—two or three times a day he would refresh himself with a glass of bromide and seltzer. Here in paradise he would stroll over to the neighborhood drugstore and have some almost every evening, to "settle his stomach" so he could sleep well. I believe, he also took two or three in the course of the day. One night his wife telephoned—her husband was breathing stertorously and she couldn't wake him. . . . He was dead when I arrived.

My friend had taken several doses of the stuff about dinner time, couldn't eat, and had retired early. About midnight, intensely cyanotic and unconscious, he died. I was not his physician—he hadn't seen a physician for a year or more—but his former doctor obligingly signed the death certificate: "heart failure" or something of the sort. I happen to believe the man suffered from chronic acetanilide poisoning and died from an overdose of acetanilide.

One of my patients, a woman about 50, suffered with chronic acetanilid poisoning as a result of constantly taking headache tablets, each tablet containing a few grains of acetanilid mixed with a little caffeine. Caffeine stimulates brain, nerves, heart and kidneys, but it is not an antidote to acetanilid poisoning. Notwithstanding her gaunt, haggard look and livid complexion, druggists kept assuring her the headache tablets were harmless and selling her this and that nostrum to strengthen her blood. Eventually she came under medical care. It took three weeks to break the acetanilid habit and nearly a year to restore fairly good health.

Nowadays, many aspirin eaters switch to tranquilizers and barbiturates which they get on prescription from reputable pharmacies. Unfortunately, when reputable pharmacies refuse to refill such prescriptions addicts can buy supplies of their favorite drugs from bootleggers.

The matriarch of a large family keeps on hand plenty of aspirin and doles it out freely whenever a relative or neighbor seems out of sorts or under the weather. This woman really believes she is doing good. I dare not tell her she is doing harm. If I ventured to do so I'm afraid all the leading doctors in her little community would assure her most positively that aspirin is harmless. They would also assure her that Brady has been repudiated by the medical profession, the cheat-food vendors, the prescription nostrum makers and the public prints, a large part of whose revenue the others contribute.

In the chapter on calcium I suggest that the peevishness and ill-humor of many persons, especially those who get insufficient exercise, is due to calcium shortage. "Calcium, if you absorb enough of it from day to day, does in a natural way what tranquilizers, sedatives, analgesics and narcotics only seem to do, if you're satisfied with half-measures," I say. I am not just a-whistling when I say you will have little or no need for such drugs, including alcohol, if you get an adequate daily ration of calcium along with enough vitamin D to insure good utilization of the calcium, 365 days in the year.

Some people become so fond of aspirin that they use it as a cure-all. With childlike credulity they take seriously the assurance of the hired hucksters that you give the stuff to children, straight or, "like a doctor's prescription," in combination with acetanilid, caffein, phenacetin (acetphetidin), bromide, aminopyrin and so on, not just for ache or pain but for "cold", tonsillitis, sore throat, fever or whatever ails your child.

Fever is not a disease. It is a sign that the body is fighting or resisting infection and therefore we should generally let it alone. A mother of fair intelligence can tell by feeling the child's forehead whether the child is feverish. Anyway, if you are going to determine by the patient's temperature whether aspirin or other medicine is to be used, it would be far better to ignore the fever.

I have always maintained and still maintain that no one, not even a trained nurse, should use a clinical thermomether or keep a record of a patient's temperature except under specific direction of the physician. A clinical thermometer in the home, some one who knows how to read it and a box of aspirin at hand can add up to a lot of mischief.

Chapter Nineteen

THEY USED TO CALL IT "RHEUMATIZ"

In that famous classic of medical literature, *The Principles and Practice of Medicine,* Dr. William Osler begins his description of each major disease by *defining* the disease, thus:

"Lobar Pneumonia.—An infectious disease characterized by inflammation of the lungs, toxemia of varying intensity, and a fever that usually terminates by crisis."

"Chronic Bronchitis.—It is the winter cough of the aged."

"Angina Pectoris.—A symptom associated with a number of morbid conditions of the heart and vessels . . . characterized by paroxysms of agonizing pain in the region of the heart, extending into the arms and neck."

But when Osler comes to *chronic rheumatism* he does not define what he is talking about—for the same reason, I suppose, that present day authors or authorities do not define what they call "the common cold"—they imply that any fool knows what a "cold" is. And so Dr. Osler merely says:

"Chronic rheumatism comes on insidiously, in persons who have passed the middle period of life. . . . It is most common among the poor, particularly washer-women, day-laborers, and those whose occupation exposes them to cold and damp."

Without disparagement to Osler's preeminence as physician and teacher 60 years ago, we have learned a little more about the nature, cause, prevention and treatment of chronic joint disability than was known in Osler's day. On the basis of this newer knowledge I beg to state that the first part of his description of chronic rheumatism is true, but the second is bunk.

Chronic joint disability, call it what you will, is NOT more prevalent among the poor, particularly washer-women, day-laborers and those who occupations expose them to cold and damp.

I often wish I could have been around, kibitzing in my irritating way, when Osler was trying to dictate his book to his faithful secretary—provided, of course, I could have used 20th century ammunition against the kind they had in the Gay Nineties. One can only conjecture how much harm Osler's preoccupation with washer-women, day-laborers and *exposure to cold and damp* has done in the world—I hate even to think about it.

It seems to me that his view of the matter was distorted by the narrowness of his field of observation. Nearly all of his experience had been gained in the wards of hospitals—where washer-women and day-laborers naturally predominated. I have a hunch that doctors in private practice see more joint disability in fairly well-to-do patients than in the poor. As for "exposure to cold and damp," if you insist on dragging that into the discussion, I had rather not argue with you—I have something more important to do with my time, namely, bowling on the green.

The association of cold and damp with "the rheumatiz" was widely accepted as obvious in Osler's time. So far as I have been able to learn no physician of standing ventured to question it until we were into the twentieth century. Likewise, as I learned the hard way, a doctor risked loss of professional reputation if he tried to teach people that so-called "colds" are communicable and have nothing to do with cold or dampness. Indeed it was because my professional reputation was shattered by my contributions to medical journals in the first decade of the century, that I had to turn to quacking it in the newspapers to provide bread and butter, shoes and stuff for my family.

In the early years of my career as a syndicated health columnist —my career was launched May 11, 1914—elderly victims of chronic joint disability used to chide me for teaching that weather, season, climate and exposure to cold and damp has nothing to do with their condition. Some of them predicted that I'd know more when I grew older and had "the rheumatiz" myself. They didn't specify how old—I'm 80 now and as reckless about exposure to cold as I am fussy about exposure to the conversation spray of persons who have the c r i. I have yet to feel the first twinge of "the rheumatiz."

If or when I become old enough to have it, as my readers predicted, I hope it won't be as painful as was the bursitis I had 30 years ago.

I was going to start repeating that story about my bursitis as an interlude here, but on reflection I had better not. It might add to the confusion of bursitis with "rheumatiz." Bursitis and rheumatism —call it "arthritis" if you prefer—have one thing in common: both are painful. I *know* bursitis is painful, and from what victims of rheumatism tell me, that must be painful too.

Although Dr. Osler did not define chronic rheumatism, what he said about it is a better definition than any present-day authority can give of "arthritis." It is notable, I think, that *The Arthritis and Rheumatism Foundation*, which issues many booklets and bulletins to press and public, has never ventured to tell how to distinguish arthritis from rheumatism—I doubt they ever will.

Some physicians writing for newspapers or magazines frankly acknowledge that "arthritis" is a misnomer, for the word means joint inflammation yet in most cases of chronic joint disability there is no sign of inflammation.

Well then, why do they exploit millions of poor souls with such a phony diagnosis? Because the customers ask for it, so to speak. I get this impression from correspondence with victims of chronic joint disability throughout the country. My correspondence with them is as confidential as they care to keep it, but I will say this much: a good many are offended when I suggest that their trouble is just old-fashioned "rheumatiz." Do I take 'em for washer-women and day-laborers?

Mind, now, I do not say genuine arthritis can't happen. In perhaps one or two cases out of a 100, joint disability is genuine arthritis, which occurs as a complication of some such infection as scarlet fever, brucellosis (undulant fever, Malta fever), tuberculosis, spotted fever (cerebrospinal meningitis), typhoid fever, gonorrhea.

Genuine arthritis differs from "rheumatiz" in onset, which is comparatively sudden, whereas rheumatism, as Dr. Osler emphasized, comes on insidiously, so gradually that it takes the victim the better part of a year to realize what ails him.

The insidious onset of rheumatism is a boon to the merchants of medicine. In the year or so it takes for the victim to find out the nature of his trouble—if he ever does find out—he or she will have spent a mint of money for miracle drugs which the merchants will "try" on their credulous customers as long as their wide-eyed faith holds out.

By this time, I imagine, some of you are wondering why I don't stow the gab and reveal the nature, cause and cure of "the rheumatiz," if I know so much more about it than other doctors do.

How come, one correspondent asked, probably looking down his nose, that you're so much more learned than the others? He went on to list certificates from no less than six boards of examiners —Medicine, Surgery, Obstetrics, Pediatrics and so on which hang on the office walls of his personal physician and demanded whether I could match 'em. Bowing and scraping I had to confess that mine number only three, to wit: a medical school diploma giving me the M. D. degree; a hospital diploma attesting satisfactory service as intern; and my license from the State of New York to practice any or all the branches mentioned and then some. Somehow I feel that this lost me his good will and that it will make him happy when all the nostrum makers and the denatured-food vendors get around to my column in the paper he reads.

Please bear with me. We will get down to brass tacks in due course. But there are a few observations it is necessary to make before we set forth the nature, cause and prevention of rheumatism —and who said anything about cure?

THE EXPERTS LOVE TO JUGGLE THE TYPES   In horse and buggy days, before the trick specialists invented "arthritis," physicians recognized two types of chronic joint disability, namely, chronic rheumatism and arthritis deformans—and they hedged on the latter by calling it "rheumatoid arthritis."

Today the experts, at least in medical journal contributions and medical textbooks, distinguish at least three types: just plain arthritis, which I gather affects people who consider themselves a cut above washer-women and day-laborers; rheumatoid arthritis, which supposedly occurs in younger persons; and osteo-arthritis, also called hypertrophic arthritis, which I confess I just don't understand—every juggler of types has his own ideas about it, and no two sets of ideas coincide.

A medical school instructor recently begged me not to introduce any new terms. He said it was difficult enough already to teach students in the two "arthritis" clinics in which he works. He said the condition I call "rheumatiz" and ascribe to degeneration of joint tissues is the degenerative type of arthritis. All I can say is I can see why it is difficult to teach medical students such balderdash.

Like a good many other doctors this man evidently cherishes the notion that arthritis means a specific condition. It doesn't. It means joint inflammation and nothing else. What joint inflammation "of the degenerative type" would mean is beyond my ken.

Degeneration, we had better explain here, is a "retrogressive pathological change in cells or tissues in consequence of which the functioning power is" (impaired or) "lost and the living substance becomes converted into an inert mass." In other words, as the cells wear out and die they are no longer replaced by new cells that carry on the same function but by fibrous, fatty or other non-functioning matter not unlike plaster-of-Paris—calcification. This calcification of body tissues, this "deposit" of calcium, is always a *consequence,* never a cause of degeneration or impairment of tissue function. It is well to get this undeniable fact through your head if you hope to prevent, retard, arrest or, I am tempted to say, cure your "rheumatiz."

EXPOSURE TO COLD AND DAMP Doctors and even ordinary folks nowadays seem less and less concerned about cold and damp, except in daydreams about the vast benefits those with "the rheumatiz" may derive from another climate—any climate far enough away from home. "Rheumatiz" or no "rheumatiz," I happen to like year-around comfort, and so I would rather live in Southern California than anywhere else in the world, for to me the climate here is more comfortable for year-round living than any other I know.

At the same time I don't believe that climate as such has anything to do with rheumatism—not even if you call it arthritis. Whatever benefit you may derive from "climate" anywhere depends entirely on how much time you spend out of doors. At best such benefit does not warrant any great sacrifices or uprooting. If you do plan to move, the wise course would be to spend a month or longer in the place where you think you want to settle before you decide whether or not to make it your permanent residence.

When I was a boy in Canandaigua, heavy woolen or red flannel underwear was *de rigueur* from Halloween to the Fourth of July, and this armor was reinforced by chest protectors, or in some cases pneumonia jackets. The pneumonia jacket was a quilted, thickly padded vest you donned perhaps in early winter, when you were threatened with a "cold" in the chest, and once they had you in it of course it could not be taken off until summer. That was doctor's order.

I am neither stoic nor insensitive to cold and damp. On the contrary, no one enjoys being nice and warm more than I do. But I do believe that the less clothing child or adult wears the better for health, provided physical comfort be the only purpose of wearing or not wearing anything. A person with low metabolism, hypothyroidism or iodine deficiency usually feels chilly when others are quite comfortable and needs and should wear warmer clothing. But this is a better solution than insisting on overheating apartment, office, shop or schoolroom regardless of the discomfort this may give normal occupants.

If you really enjoy cold showers there's no harm in the habit, but I doubt that they are of any particular benefit to health or V I T E. Certainly there is no convincing evidence that taking cold plunges or showers lessens susceptibility to c r i. As for predisposing to "rheumatiz," that's "for the birds." I say this in spite of the case I know of a Civil War veteran who, some fifty years after the battle of Shiloh, asked for and received an increase in his pension because he had slept on the damp ground one night at the time of the battle and now, as duly attested by his doctor, had "the rheumatiz" as a consequence.

Perhaps I ought to mention I was the doctor who helped the

Captain get away with it. I salved my conscience by saying the Captain *claimed* etc. etc. What could I do—here I was, the newest doctor in town, and the Captain one of the town's most respected citizens? Besides, I will stretch the truth to the breaking point any time to help a soldier's family.

DEGENERATION OF JOINT TISSUES I have the unmitigated audacity, the nerve and the gall, if you like, to say that up to now no one has discovered the nature, cause and cure of chronic joint disability, whether you call it rheumatism, chronic arthritis or just joint disability of insidious onset and long duration.

In saying this I am not unmindful of the egregious suggestion that "if the oils in your body dry out, the joints begin to creak," so what you need is a good lubricant, something to oil your joints.

Let me reiterate what I explained elsewhere: The joints of a healthy person contain no oil. They are sufficiently lubricated by the few drops of serum secreted by the serous membrane which lines the joints.

Cod liver oil is perhaps the best old time remedy for "the rheumatiz." It remains an excellent remedy for chronic joint disability, not because it is an oil or "lubricates" the joints but because it is the best natural source of vitamin D and iodine. For the same reason other foods rich or comparatively rich in vitamin D and iodine should be included in the diet of anyone with "the rheumatiz." This means plenty of butter, milk, cream, eggs, herring, sardines and canned salmon.

So much for "rheumatiz B.B." (Before Brady).

In this respect rheumatism (or "arthritis" if you prefer) is like "the common cold": Everybody talks about it but nobody tells us just what it is. For 50 years or longer, if you believe what you read in the papers, eminent specialists, scientific investigators, research experts and the like have been discovering the germ or virus of "the common cold," and with announcement of each discovery there has been almost invariably a prediction that a serum would presently be available to prevent or cure it. I have tried in vain to persuade the hunters of the elusive germ or virus to define "the common cold" so that a plodding old fogy like myself might distinguish it from specific common respiratory infections. But the medical scientists *pro tempore* loftily ignore my plea—and besides, they imply, everyone knows what a common cold is.

Those who exploit the credulous public with remedies or treatments purporting to be good for "arthritis" have nothing to say about its nature or cause. Why should they commit themselves when most of their customers won't even ask?

The only medical textbook that defines chronic joint disability in the way such a textbook should is that quaint tome of Osler's which somebody once called "the doctor's bible." Osler alone described the morbid anatomy or pathology of chronic joint disability, as *degeneration of joint tissues,* although he called it chronic rheumatism.

Latter-day specialists prefer to keep people as ignorant and confused as possible, for that makes it easy to sell 'em course after course of treatment with modern miracle drugs as fast as these are "accepted" by organized medicine.

Obviously I am a skeptic regarding medication for joint disability, yet only four or five years ago I fell hard for a drug called butazolidin. I actually saw a patient—not my own—who had been crippled with what her doctor called "arthritis" get up and dance about the room after two days of butazolidin. I was amazed. I wanted to tell everybody about it and naturally did so in my newspaper column. But alas, a few days later the patient was as badly crippled as ever. So I wrote about that too. Soon afterward I learned that the medicine had proved dangerous and for a while I lived in fear, but, thank the Lord, there were no repercussions and I concluded that readers had not been able to get any of the medicine to try, since a prescription was necessary.

The nature of chronic joint disability, of insidious onset and long duration, the condition I call *RHEUMATIZ* is—let's face it— *degeneration of joint tissues*.

If you ask me about arthritis, I can only advise you to consult a physician.

If you ask me about rheumatism, I don't know what you're talking about.

If you ask me about *RHEUMATIZ* I'll tell you it is degeneration of the joint tissues due to *nutritional deficiency* through the years from childhood up to the present, and that it is chiefly a calcium, vitamin D, iodine and vitamin B deficiency.

There's no more to tell about the nature and cause of insidiously developing joint disability of long standing. If you want to know more about it, turn back to the chapters where I discuss the relation of food and nutrition to degeneration in general and "the rheumatiz" in particular.

The concept of chronic joint disability I present here is not something I picked out of the air. It is a conviction that came from a professional lifetime study of the question. I am not promoting any remedy or cure. I merely recommend a regimen, a way of life to prevent, relieve or, if adopted in time and consistently followed for life, perhaps even cure "the rheumatiz." This last claim I hesitate to make. But I am emboldened to speak of cure by numerous reports I have received from victims who declare they really are cured and back at the jobs their "rheumatiz" had forced them to give up.

The regimen is not medicine you can sample for a few weeks. Rather it is a way of life to follow from childhood to old age. "Rheumatiz" is not the only disability the regimen prevents, postpones or alleviates. But I'm afraid to mention other degenerations the regimen prevents, lest some half-informed readers think I really have lost most of my marbles.

THE REGIMEN FOR RHEUMATIZ The regimen is basically quite simple, yet difficult to follow regularly nowadays. The essential features are adequate daily rations of calcium, vitamin D, iodine and vitamin B complex.

An adequate daily ration of calcium for a sedentary person past the middle period of life is supplied by one and a half pints of milk or for a growing child or physically active youth not less than a quart.

You can get an adequate ration of vitamin D, iodine and vitamin A from two tablespoonfuls, or one ounce, of cod liver oil daily.

You can get all the vitamin D required for good metabolism of calcium in the body from exposing as much skin surface as possible to sunshine or skyshine at every opportunity. In that way you give the invisible, ultraviolet rays of sunlight a chance to act upon sterols in the skin to generate viosterol, vitamin D.

You can get all the vitamin B complex required for good nutrition from plain wheat. This is the most difficult part of the regimen. It is difficult for two reasons: First, because the commercial milling interests do not want people to use wheat as a staple—they want to sell refined white flour; second, because people today haven't time to fuss with cooking and baking, they prefer to get their food ready-to-eat or ready to "pop in the oven" so they can devote themselves to bridge, movies, TV, cocktail parties etc.

I have been dropped by many large newspapers at the insistence of the refined white flour interests. "Kill Brady or else," they say. The cheat-food vendors do not like me very well, even though they censor my column ruthlessly. They know I send a free pamphlet, *Wheat to Eat,* to anyone who asks for it and provides a stamped, self-addressed envelope; and that this pamphlet has been instrumental in restoring plain wheat as a staple of everyday diet in many homes.

From reports my followers send me I conclude that the most important part of the "rheumatiz" regimen is an *optimal daily ration of calcium and vitamin D*. By optimal I mean an amount twice or three times that which nutrition authorities consider essential for preventing deficiency disease. In other words, in addition to a *high calcium diet,* you would do well to supplement it with calcium and vitamin D in other forms, as for istance four Calcicaps or two Calciwafers daily. Often this supplement may be discontinued after four to six months if improvement is satisfactory; and the diet may be varied somewhat. But you had better continue giving preference to high calcium foods for the rest of your life, being particularly careful to drink at least one and a half pints of milk each day the year around.

But this is only half the regimen. If you are either developing or already suffering from chronic joint disability, there are two other nutritional deficiencies to correct. These are B-complex deficiency and iodine deficiency. Both are important factors of good nutrition. Up to the present, doctors and folks have learned little about them —little truth, that is, with a lot of fiction and conjecture.

A Chicago woman reported that after following the "rheumatiz" regimen three months she got wonderful relief from her "arthritis" of several years' standing. Housework had been a real problem, but now she could get down and scrub floors without any trouble.

For six months a New York man followed the regimen and then, at age 64, began to feel almost as good as when he started work as a letter-carrier at the age of 40. He was so much improved, in fact, and was able to resume work on the old job.

An Ohio woman says she has followed the regimen for about six months. She had been so crippled up with joint disability that she was quite helpless. She declares she is as good as ever now.

"I didn't really expect much improvement," writes a New Jersey woman, "but to my surprise, after five or six weeks on the regimen, the swelling and pain in various joints started to diminish and soon I was able to get in and out of bed without trouble. It is wonderful to get about the house and yard again. . . ."

"This is the first winter," writes a Massachusetts reader, "in six or seven years that I haven't had a bad spell of rheumatiz. I shall certainly continue the regimen from now on."

A Texas woman who could hardly get out of bed mornings hasn't had an ache or pain for the past six months and she thanks God for the rheumatiz regimen.

Last winter was the first winter a Michigan woman's husband has been comfortable, no pains or "growing old" aches, thanks to the regimen.

A Pennsylvania woman says she was unable to even move around the house without pain until she had followed the regimen for a month. Now she even gets out to the market with comfort.

An Ontario woman gradually got so stiff in all her joints that she couldn't get out of bed or, once she sat up, couldn't lift her feet to finish dressing. She adopted the regimen for rheumatiz and got some relief inside a month. No aches or pains at all now. She is very grateful.

"You have no idea how my health has improved since I went on the rheumatiz regimen," reports a Minnesota woman. "After four years in and out of hospitals, loss of work, medications galore, not to mention the suffering I experienced with so-called 'arthritis,' I learned about your regimen. Now I'm feeling my old self again. I don't know what would have become of me. . . ."

I dunno—maybe printing these testimonials will make me qualify for a blooming quack, but I don't care. I just thought it might help to persuade some "arthritis" victims to take a more sensible view of their joint disability.

Chapter Twenty

ALCOHOL IS A NARCOTIC

In the Victorian era alcohol, preferably in the form of brandy—though gin, Scotch or Bourbon would do in a pinch—was virtually a panacea, good for everything from swooning to snakebite.

According to Webster, the Victorian era ended officially in 1901 —the year I was admitted to the medical profession. By the time the profession realized its mistake I was practicing in Penn Yan.

Three years after the close of the era, in 1904, the tenth edition of Hare's *Practical Therapeutics* was published. In the chapter on alcohol the author said:

Alcohol never acts as a true stimulant to the brain, the spinal cord, or the nerves. On the contrary, its dominant influence is depressant. . . . Alcohol is in no sense a true stimulant to the circulation. If the dose is large enough to cause any appreciable change in the circulation, it is in the nature of depression rather than stimulation. . . .

The chief uses of alcohol are as a rapidly acting stimulant in all forms of cardiac failure due to shock or poisons . . . additional conditions in which alcohol is indicated are fainting, snakebite, surgical shock and wasting diseases.

I wished heartily that I had my money back—I had plunked down $3.75 for the book. When I questioned the author about his badly contradictory statements, he calmly answered:

"It is quite conceivable that alcohol acts as a stimulant upon other functions of which, as yet, we know very little, as, for example, the ability of the body to resist infection."

That tore it. It wasn't so much the $3.75, though that wasn't hay in 1905. It was a disheartening feeling that the profession had let me down. Ever since, I have been at odds with one or another element and only the other day one doctor—it would do no good to identify him—protested in the Public Forum of a New England newspaper:

"But why do you continue to permit Dr. Brady to publish this nonsense . . . anyone who advocates delivering babies at home. . . . Find someone to write articles who does not have a chip on his shoulder and is not 'mad at the medical profession'."

Correction: I'm not mad at the *entire* medical profession all at one time. I'm mad at the trick specialists one day, the "clinic" racketeers the next, the AMA another day, and so on. And I wasn't even mad over Dr. Hare's defection—just saddened. For I had worshipped Hare, placing him on a pedestal alongside of Osler. I still revere his memory: he was a great teacher. I have yet to see a finer textbook of therapeutics than my precious tenth edition of Hare.

What does make me really mad, though, is the way the merchants of medicine make like specialists, prescribing medicines by proprietary or trade names so they will cost patients three or four times as much as when they are prescribed by generic or chemical names. I also object to doctors participating in such gouging of the public, though I do not mean to imply they collect a percentage from pharmacist or manufacturer. Sometimes they simply don't know enough about the drug to give its generic name. All they do know is what the detail men tell them.

I may be wrong, but I confess it beats me how doctors can take some of the inconsistencies of modern medicine without batting an eyelash. Hare, for instance, not just a physician but a teacher, a professor in a great medical school and a recognized authority, first asserts that alcohol never acts as a true stimulant to the brain, nerves or circulation, then says its chief use is as a rapidly acting stimulant in heart failure, shock or fainting. I was saddened by all this. But the man's rejoinder to my slightly querulous complaint, which he made September 21, 1906 (I have the letter pasted in the book), was even more disturbing. In Hare's time no one knew anything about the ability of the body to resist infection—beyond taking a leucocyte (phagocyte, white blood corpuscle) count, and we know almost as little about "resistance" today. That is to say, all our imposing references to "lowered resistance," "maintaining good resistance" and the like are pure hooey. There's not a scintilla of scientific evidence that alcohol or other medicine "acts as a stimulant" to resistance.

At the moment I am reminded of other inconsistencies in the views and teachings of medical authorities, inconsistencies that tend to make a student cynical if not skeptical. It is bad enough that we must be constantly alert to commercially inspired subversion; we must also be vigilant against ust plain poor judgment.

Perhaps Prof. Hare's teachings about alcohol were calculated to please everybody, whereas my teachings are calculated to irritate everybody except a few teetotalers. After all, if the truth hurts it's not my fault.

Alcohol in any dose and any circumstance is a narcotic.

Alcohol is a depressant to the heart, the nerves, the brain and the circulation.

When we say alcohol we mean beer, wine or liquor. Beer is four to six per cent alcohol. Wine is approximately 16 per cent, whiskey or brandy 50 per cent alcohol. Gin and vodka are practically straight alcohol, which is a mixture of alcohol (48.9 per cent by volume) in water—this is the alcohol, officially called Diluted Alcohol in the U.S. Pharmacopoeia, used in medicine. Absolutely pure alcohol (100 per cent strength) is rarely obtainable. "Deodorized alcohol" or "cologne spirit" is 94.9 per cent (by volume) alcohol. Most gin is pure alcohol, water and flavoring, mainly essence of juniper berries.

In the seventeenth century, says that interesting and instructive volume, *The Commonsense Book of Drinking,* by Leon D. Adams, a Dutch professor named Sylvius discovered that the nauseous taste of the crudely distilled spirits of that era could be masked successfully with fragrant juniper berries and thereby made palatable. This was the original gin.

Gin became important in America in the prohibition era when people bought alcohol from bootleggers, glycerin and juniper oil from drugstores and mixed them together to make bathtub gin. Juniper flavored alcohol in potent Martinis has been a status symbol of the party-throwing set ever since.

Mr. Adams respects the freedom of the individual to drink so long as he doesn't harm or annoy others, but he punctures the pretense of the drinker who displays his sophistication by insisting on only this or that brand of gin in his Martini cocktail. These smart drinkers are just as silly about vodka. For instance, six expert professional tasters tried and failed to distinguish a well-known brand of 80-proof vodka from ordinary grain alcohol diluted with water down to the same strength. Vodka, says Mr. Adams, is nothing more nor less than watered alcohol. I'm afraid the snob boozers will be indignant about this.

Like Mr. Adams I respect the freedom of the adult to drink. But to my sober mind the pomp and ceremony with which crapulous drinkers endeavor to make their tippling polite and respectable is childish, hollow and tiresome. The sight of a bartender or a host doing the cocktail shaking act makes me long for a wet dishrag with which to swat the guy.

Then there is the toast business. Even if you do not regard it as asinine, tell me this: Why is water, coffee, lemonade, milk or pop not as appropriate for a toast as liquor? And what kind of host or hostess fails to provide for or embarrasses the guest who happens to be a teetotaler?

The author of *The Prodigal Shepherd,* Father Pfau, tells quite frankly how he became an alcoholic. As a newly ordained priest assigned to a post as assistant to the pastor of a large parish he was a guest at the home of an affable man of means and there met some pleasant people. They seemed to enjoy their drinks without getting out of line, so after a while Father Pfau decided he'd try something stronger than lemonade. For a long time after he had become addicted and all his associates knew of his drinking, Father Pfau kept insisting to himself that he was not an alcoholic. Indeed he never did admit it until he joined Alcoholics Anonymous. Now, as all members do, he begins his talks to groups by saying: "I am an alcoholic." The idea is, once an alcoholic, always an alcoholic, even though you never again take a drink. This is part of the A.A.

philosophy—a philosophy which has restored a good many alcoholics to sobriety.

The kind of wrong thinking which kept Father Pfau from acknowledging that he was an alcoholic keeps too many alcoholics from attending group meetings regularly once they have attended one or two. They persist in flattering themselves that *they* are a cut above the drunkards they see there and so they discontinue attendance.

It is thinking typical of the early stages of alcoholism. Everybody has heard the incipient alcoholic assert vehemently that he knows what he is doing, he can take it or let it alone, he can stop drinking any time he wants to stop and so doesn't need advice or help from anybody.

ALCOHOL IS A NARCOTIC It is the cheapest and most readily available narcotic. The amount of alcohol in even one cocktail is sufficient to slow reaction time and decrease reflex activity, even though the individual may not seem intoxicated in the popular sense. This is physiological fact, not just my notion. An automobile driver, a railroad engineer or a pilot who takes just one drink before going on duty or while on duty endangers both his own life and the lives of passengers, even though witnesses may testify he is not intoxicated.

To my way of thinking—call me a puritan if you will—admission or proof that a driver or pilot had taken just one drink should be sufficient to convict in any accident case. The arbitrary determination of intoxication by measuring the quantity of alcohol in the blood or in the exhaled air is plain miscarriage of justice.

Here are some of the effects of a small dose of alcohol on performance:

(1) Typesetters are slower and make more mistakes.
(2) Typists make more errors.
(3) Pianists strike more wrong notes.
(4) Marksmanship with pistol or rifle is inferior.
(5) Needle threading becomes more difficult.
(6) Sight and hearing are less keen.

(7) The sense of touch, as measured by the delicate es-
thesiometer, is impaired.

(8) Automobile drivers are a fraction of a second slower in
braking when an unexpected obstacle looms in front
of them.

All of these effects are the effects of a *narcotic*. They are practically the same as those produced by morphine or heroin.

But the manufacture and sale of alcoholic beverages bring the
government enormous tax revenue, so the government can't be
too hard on big business. But you and I pay the tax, at the state and
municipal level—and then we have to maintain the hospitals, jails
and police force that alcohol makes necessary, to say nothing of
condoning the poverty, suffering, shame and sorrow it brings to
our children.

Riffle the pages of any popular magazine, particularly in holiday
season, and the elaborate, costly beer, wine and liquor ads will
convince you that alcohol is indeed big business. I know of a man
not quite forty who regularly went on a bender two or three times
a year, to the distress of his family, business associates and friends.
Yet between binges he drank little or nothing. In a lucid interval he
once tried to explain why he did it. But the best he could do was,
"At times I drink to excess because I feel the need of a stimulant,
or rather I just want to feel better."

"Need of a stimulant" is a vague way of admitting consciousness
or inferiority. This inferiority is not necessarily any specific thing,
like awareness of lack of education, social position or good breed-
ing, or self-consciousness about personal appearance. Rather it
means, I think, awareness of imperfect or poor health.

Every one consciously or unconsciously compares his own health
with the health of people around him who enjoy or seem to enjoy
vitality. Unfortunately some persons with this inferiority feeling
imagine they can dispel the feeling, at least for an hour or two, by
taking a few drinks. The alcohol makes them, for the time being,
less conscious of what they consider their own shortcomings—and
they childishly call it being stimulated.

It is because alcohol is a depressant to the higher consciousness
that for an hour or so the individual becomes less conscious or

aware of his inferiority. Alcohol depresses or renders less efficient every function of the body.

When I was a member of the Chapel Street gang in Canandaigua I suffered for a while because a certain Mrs. Hawkshaw came along one day, inspected me critically and told mother she'd never raise *that one*. She diagnosed my trouble as "worms." I guess Mrs. Hawkshaw had the goods on me—I had black hair, freckles and those telltale white lines around the gills. I can still taste the horrible worm medicine they made me take. Aside from that I have enjoyed excellent health all my life. I enjoy it now—so much that I hate to lose any time from enjoyment of life. But that is not the only reason why I'm a teetotaler. A more cogent reason is that Mother was a member of the W.C.T.U. More about that anon.

Although I practice total abstinence as a matter of health, principle and example, I can understand why a person who suffers from malnutrition, that is, impairment of health due to nutritional deficiency, may feel the craving for a drink. The poor sap is just too dumb to correct his faulty diet, improve his nutritional condition and build up his VITE.

I am not trying to tell you that anyone who craves alcohol is going to lose that craving merely by supplementing his everyday diet with adequate daily rations of the vitamins and minerals of which our refined American eating habits have robbed him. Abundant supplies of calcium, phosphorus and iodine, of vitamin B_1 or thiamin, vitamin B_2 or riboflavin and vitamin D—or eating 6 Ray-D tablets daily—won't cure an alcoholic overnight. But I am convinced that some such nutritional improvement will enable many an *incipient* alcoholic to learn to say "no, thank you"—and mean it.

If you are in A-one nutritional condition—if you have VITE, that is, and feel fine and dandy, you won't need alcohol, stimulants, aspirin, tonic, tranquilizers, bracers, barbiturates or any other dope. If you have VITE you will not drink—unless you've inherited some mental defect. You will find yourself a total abstainer, first because alcohol can add nothing to your sense of well-being, secondly because it is your duty to abstain in order to be an example for the young.

Even if I'd had unlimited choice I don't believe I could have chosen better parents than God gave me, and I thank Him for my parents every day of my life. For one thing, they asked all of us children to take the pledge not to use alcohol or tobacco until we were 21. All four of us kept the pledge, which we had taken at the age of eight to ten years.

Most of the children in the neighborhood where we grew up not only never took the pledge but evinced their contempt for such sissy prohibition by smoking cigarettes and, as children will do, spitting through their teeth. Later, when they got along into teen age, some of these children demonstrated their manliness by drinking, first beer, a popular brand of which was brewed in the village (some readers will remember Canandaigua Ale), and finally whiskey. A few of these show-offs never reached high school but they did make police court and jail.

I call them show-offs—that characterization applies equally well to a large section of adult drinkers too, drinkers who never get any- where in the world except to divorce court, drinkers like the ones in *The Common Sense Book of Drinking* who couldn't distinguish vodka from ordinary alcohol watered to 80-proof.

I'm afraid nowadays most parents no longer ask their children to take the pledge, either because they are themselves too fond of drinking or because they are just too wishy-washy to take a stand on anything. Some of these flabby characters even argue that it is morally wrong to ask a child to take the pledge—every child should decide for himself whether to drink or not. On the same basis parents should leave it to the child whether he shall accept or re- ject the Ten Commandments.

In the years I have been pleading for temperance as an elemen- tary principle of health and happiness I have been dismayed by what seems to be a growing disinclination of ministers, priests and rabbis to ask children to take the pledge. I am happy to note how- ever that a great many readers tell me they took the pledge when they were confirmed and have kept it for life. We know of course that booze is big business in Yankeeland, but after all. . . .

When I think of the pledge, I think of the Women's Christian Temperance Union, of which Mother was a member. The W.C.T.U. was and still is the main support of the pledge. Judging by the ex- perience of the Brady boys, all gone now with one exception, it had a far-reaching influence, equalled only by that of our grade-school teacher, the sainted Miss Lutie Berner whom I mentioned earlier in the book. Miss Lutie's influence, lined up behind that of our parents, was additional assurance that we would never break the pledge.

Whatever the excuse or occasion for drinking may be, you must remember that alcohol is always a narcotic, never a stimulant and never a tonic. Still, confronted with minor or major emergency, any ninnyhammer can find in folklore or in medical literature justification for giving a victim a shot of liquor.

Contemplating the frightful amount of crime, disease, deprivation, cruelty to children, divorce, degradation, misery and unhappiness chargeable to drinking, I like to think what a boon it would be to America if every child at the age of ten would take the pledge not to drink—and keep the pledge for life.

Chapter Twenty-one

PLAIN TALK ABOUT YOUR HEART

Bartlett's, Stevenson's and other books give hundreds of quotations that refer to the heart, all of them poetic or figurative. Modern books filled with four-letter words and plays dealing with prostitution and homosexuality indulge in no such circumlocutions. But even though they may sound coldly clinical, they still do not give the public the anatomical or physiological facts.

The arteries that supply the heart itself—the heart is a hollow muscle—spread out over its base in a manner that to the ancients suggested a crown, and so these arteries were named the coronary arteries. Unfortunately in England in former times the officer who investigated sudden, unexplained fatalities was an officer of the crown and came to be called the crowner or coroner. This coincidence sometimes makes for confusion.

It is beyond the scope of this chapter to discuss coronary occlusion, coronary thrombosis or coronary spasm, known as angina pectoris, further than to say that an attack may be so mild it is not recognized as a heart attack or severe enough to require absolute rest for two or three months. This doesn't necessarily mean confinement to bed. It has been found that coronary patients as a rule do better if after the first week they are allowed to sit in an armchair for about half an hour in the morning and again in the evening, perhaps even longer if the patient is more comfortable in a chair.

The purpose of treatment of any kind of heart trouble is to maintain or increase the supply of oxygen through the blood to the heart muscle. Rest makes more oxygen available, the heart muscle gets the oxygen the voluntary muscles would use up if they were working. At a later stage of successful treatment exercise, whether moderate, graduated or gradually increasing, increases the absorption of oxygen, and the damaged heart benefits from it, as if from inhalations of oxygen from a tank. Indeed, oxygen inhalations are a routine part of the treatment of coronary thrombosis, to relieve pain and other distress and speed recovery and convalescence. Many good physicians now advise patients who have had one coronary or anginal attack to keep on hand or carry in pocket or handbag a small tank of oxygen to inhale whenever a seizure impends.

The best possible medicine for anyone with heart and/or artery trouble, in my judgment, is a brisk walk—neither a loll nor stroll —of from half a block to two or three miles twice daily. It may well take months to graduate from half a block to three miles of oxygen on the hoof, but as long as the exercise is moderate and not really tiring it is fine for health.

One chap about 48 or 50, who had one or maybe more than one coronary bout apparently thought he would have to walk on eggs the rest of his life. Nearly every day his chauffeur brought him to the bowling green, where he would sit watching the game. Then his chauffeur-nurse would carefully help him back to his car. I have a queer sense of humor—I had to laugh at the poor guy. In time I began to work on him. I assured him that bowling was just what he needed to complete his recovery. "Believe me, Doctor, I wish I could—" "Don't give me that hoofla," I told him. "Don't you want to get back on the job?" "More than anything in the world, but. . . ." Finally I told him I'd certainly bowl if I were in his place, and suggested that he tell his physician I said so. Presently the poor fellow began to bowl. It did my heart good to see how much good it did his heart and his outlook on life.

There are too many misguided souls, men and women, walking on eggs—if they walk at all. Following such a somber way of life tends to weaken any heart.

One man who had been invalided for several months with coronary thrombosis later took up the sport of flying. He flew across the Atlantic and skiied at an Alpine resort. Another who recovered from coronary thrombosis later ran in a Marathon race in South Africa. Not that I suggest such strenuous sport or any game or activity involving great strain or effort; this is just to point out that graduated exercise, under continuing observation by the physician, is at least as important as rest and medication in the treatment of any kind of heart disease.

What the doctor who knows his business has in mind when advising or treating a patient with heart disease is the *reserve power* of the heart. More about this later.

THE NATURE OF C.V.D. Arteriosclerosis (hardening of the arteries), myocarditis (slow heart muscle failure, degenerative changes in the heart), angina pectoria, chronic interstitial nephritis (Bright's disease) and apoplexy (stroke or shock of paralysis) are various manifestations of the condition known as cardiovascular disease or degeneration, which we designate for brevity C.V.D.

Of course arteriosclerosis is the fundamental process in C.V.D. and it is circumstantial whether it affects chiefly the aorta and the coronary arteries which supply blood to the heart itself, the general circulation, the terminal arteries in the brain, or the arterioles in the kidneys.

Cardiovascular degeneration or disease begins in the intima or lining membrane of the artery, is a nutritional condition primarily, and in the majority of cases becomes established after a more or less prolonged period of hypertension or high blood pressure.

Predominance of non-protective foods (foods from which most of the natural vitamins and minerals have been removed) in everyday diet is a factor of the degenerative changes that constitute cardiovascular disease. Restoring the natural vitamins and minerals to the diet, either by following a corrective protective diet or by daily supplementing ordinary diet with the necessary vitamins and minerals, tends to reverse these degenerative changes and bring about regeneration, and so we call such a regimen a regeneration or rejuvenation regimen. It is described in detail in "The 7 Keys to Vite."

Besides nutritional deficiencies, other contributing causes of C.V.D. in the opinion of good medical authorities are the toxins of pneumonia, typhoid fever and other infectious diseases; and alcohol, tobacco, lead, syphilis and *over-eating*.

Finally, the inheritance of poor material in the arteries is a favorite hypothetical cause of C.V.D. Dr. Osler had a good deal of reverence for this theory. Today we take a less fatalistic view of the matter. How long a man will live depends not so much upon the quality of arteries or material for arteries he was born with as on the way he lives. Prevention of premature old age and prolongation of youth is not a vascular, but a hygienic question. This is the trend of modern medical thought, based on newer knowledge of physiology and nutrition. The older view was based largely on post-mortem study, morbid anatomy. The present view is based on the study of function, animal experimentation, human life. The old time doctor was easy-going about wine, liquor, brandy and gin. He couldn't see much harm in alcohol until he had the patient's liver or kidney preserved in a jar of it. The modern practitioner says, "Practice total abstinence or else."

The unrestricted use of cathartics, especially saline cathartics, salts, mineral aperients or fortified mineral waters, is, in my opinion, a common contributing cause of C.V.D. for I believe all this interferes with the normal assimilation and retention of calcium.

VALVULAR INCOMPETENCE   Provided the heart itself, consisting mainly of involuntary muscle, is well nourished, and has an unhampered supply of blood through the coronary arteries, and provided that the blood brings the quantity and quality of nutriment required, its functional efficiency or competence to maintain good circulation under varying circumstances of rest, work, play or strain will depend upon the state of the heart valves.

In order to understand what valvular disease or incompetence or leakage means one must know that there are four chambers in the heart. As the blood circulates, first is the left auricle into which freshly oxygenated or purified blood comes through the large pulmonary veins from the lungs. From the left auricle the blood passes through the mitral valve into the left ventricle (during diastole) in the interval between the contractions or beats of the heart. When the heart beats, the mitral valve closes, preventing return of blood from the ventricle, and the blood is pumped out into the great artery or aorta through the aortic valve. Following this contraction or systole, during diastole (the rest interval between contractions) the aortic valve is closed so no blood can return to the ventricle from the aorta, but instead the elasticity of the great artery propels the blood along through the smaller arteries. Eventually the blood reaches the smallest arteries, called arterioles, visible only through microscope. Then it passes into the capillary spaces where interchange of oxygen and carbon dioxide occur.

TEST YOUR CAPILLARY CIRCULATION   Capillary means resembling a hair. The capillaries of the body, however, are not tubes or vessels at all, but just spaces between the cells through which the blood seeps as water seeps through sand. What are commonly but inaccurately called "capillary vessels" are actually arterioles. Arterioles have walls and are blood vessels; capillaries are not.

It takes the blood approximately 23 seconds or 28 heart beats to make one complete circuit of the cardiovascular system. The blood travels slowest in the capillary areas—that is, in the tissues where the oxygen is passed over to the tissue cells and the carbon dioxide picked up to be carried back to the lungs.

You may observe capillary circulation by noticing the blanching of the skin just below the base of the finger nail when you draw your thumb across the area so as to squeeze the blood out of it; and the number of seconds required for the return of the normal flush is an index of the efficiency of your capillary circulation and your general circulation as well. In a healthy person the normal flush returns within three or four seconds. In one in the early stage of cardiovascular degeneration—say thrombo-angitis from excessive smoking—the blanching remains longer, perhaps six or eight seconds.

The capillary area between the arterioles on the one side and the smallest veins, the venules, on the other, may be regarded as a lake with 600 to 800 times greater cross section area than the stream itself. Thus the velocity of movement or flow is naturally slower there. The reduced velocity has advantages, for it is here that the interchange of gases, nutritive materials and waste products takes place between blood and tissues.

From the capillary "lake" the blood passes along through the smallest veins, the venules, and on into larger veins, finally reaching the heart. It enters the right auricle through the great vein, the vena cava. From the right auricle it passes through the tricuspid valve into the right ventricle, and from the right ventricle through the pulmonary valve into the pulmonary artery which conveys the blood to the lungs. Again it passes through the capillary area in the lungs where it gives up its carbon dioxide and is freshly oxygenated—changed from venous to arterial blood. Then it is returned through the mitral valve into the left ventricle, and is finally pumped into the great artery or aorta through the aortic valve.

Although primary cause of valvular trouble may be acute, the victim generally is not aware that there is anything wrong until symptoms of valvular leakage manifest themselves and bring the patient under medical observation.

The usual cause of valvular disease is endocarditis, inflammation of the lining membrane of the heart. This is a complication of such illnesses as acute infectious arthritis ("inflammatory rheumatism, rheumatic fever"), acute tonsillitis, scarlet fever, or chorea of St. Vitus' dance. Unfortunately, as it causes no pain or other immediate alarming symptoms it may remain unrecognized until some time subsequent to the illness when impairment of the circulation becomes evident.

MOST ENDOCARDITIS PASSES UNRECOGNIZED   The popular notion of "Rheumatism of the heart" is a vague one associated with some dreadful pain around the heart. Actually when damage to the heart occurs as a complication or result of acute infectious arthritis no pain or other distress marks the occurrence. Indeed, unless the physician examines the heart daily in the course of the illness, even he may not be aware that endocarditis has developed until weeks or months, even years after the original illness, when circulatory deficiency due to valvular damage becomes manifest.

What happens is that some of the bacteria responsible for the arthritis, or perhaps only tonsillitis, scarlet fever, chorea or septic sore throat, lodge on the lining of the heart and set up an inflammation there. If this happens to be an area covering a heart valve, the exudate or "vegetations" associated with the inflammation, or the subsequent contraction of scar tissue may distort the valve slightly so that it no longer closes the orifice completely. Thence some back-flow or leakage of blood occurs with each heart beat.

While there is no pain or other distress pointing to the heart, and indeed no indication of heart mischief in most instances, if the physician had the patient under close observation he might make a fairly accurate diagnosis of acute endocarditis.

This being a health lesson, we shall not suggest symptoms of valvular disease, further than to say that the chief reason why any form of valvular disease is a handicap is that it decreases the margin of reserve power in the heart. In other words it renders a person less capable of coping with exertion or strain which calls for extra work by the heart.

NATURAL BREATHING IMPROVES CIRCULATION   The pur-pose of breathing is to supply oxygen to the blood and to blow off the carbon dioxide which the blood brings back to the lungs from the functioning muscles, organs, glands or tissues. One of the main purposes of circulation is to carry oxygen to the cells of the body and return the products of oxidation or metabolism, from the cells of muscles, organs, glands and tissues to the excretory organs (lungs, kidneys, intestine, liver and skin) for disposal. So it is clear that breathing and circulation are both concerned with oxygenation and there can be no serious disturbance or impairment of the one without involving the other.

This little lesson in physiology is of practical value to people who consider themselves well. It should interest, also, people who are subject to valvular heart trouble, myocarditis, or angina pectoris and those with high or low blood pressure, cardiovascular degen-eration, arteriosclerosis, insomnia, poor circulation, unaccountable languor, easy fatigue or other manifestations of anoxia which people so readily ascribe to "neurasthenia," whatever that may be.

Whatever ails you, the chances are you know neither how to breathe naturally nor how good it is for you to practice breathing that way—unless you have already studied the first part of this book.

ANOXIA AND HEART FAILURE   Insufficient oxygen delivered
to the cells, tissues or organs of the body—anoxia, as doctors call it
—explains all the symptoms of heart disease, whether it be valvular
leakage, angina pectoris or chronic myocarditis (slow heart muscle
failure). Complete deprivation of oxygen, cellular asphyxia, is the
cause of death in all cases of heart disease that terminate fatally.
Valvular disease is seldom fatal, however. A person with a valvular
leakage may, if he knows his handicap, recognizes his limitations
and lives within them, enjoy a longer life than the average.

Comparatively slight anoxia, as mentioned earlier, is probably
accountable for otherwise inexplicable aviation disasters attributed
to "pilot error." Among the effects of moderate oxygen want are
dulling of senses and intellect without the person being aware of it,
lowering of powers of sight, hearing, memory, judgment, irrational
ideas, uncontrolled outbursts of emotion and disturbed muscular
coordination. Such effects occur in anoxia from fever, pneumonia
and septicemia, as well as in chronic or moderate carbon monoxide
anoxia and in high flying or mountain sickness. They occur, too,
in heart disease—any kind of organic heart disease in which the
heart's reserve power is so reduced that circulation fails to supply
enough oxygen to satisfy the demands of the patient's way of living.

You see, a normal heart has power, say from A to E for the
ordinary requirements of sedentary life, moderate work or play,
and power from E to K which it can put forth in an emergency.
The E to K power is reserve power. Now suppose a valvular lesion
develops, and with each heart beat a portion of the blood leaks
back through the damaged valve. In order to still pump enough
blood into the arteries the heart must pump more at each beat than
the normal quantity to compensate for the backflow. It does this by
drawing on the reserve power. Therefore a heart with a valvular in-
sufficiency has to use the power, say from A to G even when at
rest, and has a correspondingly limited reserve to put forth in an
emergency, only from G to K.

This margin of reserve power is the determining factor in the
prognosis of not only valvular trouble but every other form of
heart disease. Husbanding reserve power by REST or increasing it
by GRADUATED EXERCISE are prime factors in the treatment
of heart disease.

THE STRENGTH OF THE HEART During the rapid growth and development from the age of ten to 18 years the heart, like other muscles, is susceptible to strain. Most intelligent people understand this and deal accordingly with growing children. But parents of high school boys are frequently either too ignorant or too negligent to offer objection, or even to ask the opinion of the family physician, when the sporting gents of the town invade the school, thrust aside qualified physical instructors and pick the boys they deem likely material for the football team. This schoolboy imitation of the university man's game gives the less wholesome element a prestige in the eyes of the youngsters subversive of true education.

The process of training, or "getting wind," involves gradual increase in the capability of the heart, particularly the right side which pumps blood to the lungs. In order to excel as a runner, wrestler, boxer, football player or oarsman, it is essential that one have an enlarged heart with enormously widened reserve power, for the heart must perform far more than its normal physiological work during such severe exertion.

"Getting second wind" is chiefly a question of the heart's reserve power. During sustained exertion the heart dilates or becomes overfilled and the breathlessness of air-hunger manifests itself first as anxiety and then as distress; at this stage (perhaps the third quarter in a mile run) the reserve power of the heart begins to be effective, and the increased volume of blood pumped to the straining muscles brings the oxygen they demand. The dilatation is overcome and the athlete experiences sudden relief from the agony of breathlessness. The diaphragm and belly muscles function more freely and the breathing is amplified.

Of course, this is not acute heart failure. Acute dilatation of the heart means that the one or more chambers of the heart become stretched, overfilled with blood, fail to empty completely during heart-beat, or systole. This is a *normal* occurrence during any unusual or violent exertion, particularly in the right ventricle which pumps blood to the lungs. With rest, the heart recovers, provided the effort or strain has not been too great or the heart has not been defective to begin with. Sometimes in these circumstances the heart suffers a strain from which it recovers slowly, or never completely, so that the victim may be thereafter unable to undertake any severe exertion or endure any physical strain.

Something like that happens to a good many schoolboys who play football. In their 'teens boys are poorly equipped to attempt the severe endurance contests which men of university age may safely withstand.

It is because strenuous athletic training necessarily produces enlargement of the heart that physicians who have studied the problem advise against such precocious affectations as football in high school. Training for football, if properly carried out under the supervision of a physician, is not injurious to men of university age. It is a dangerous thing for boys in their 'teens. At that period of life a boy's heart is taxed to supply the oxygen his rapidly growing and developing cells, tissues and organs require. To permit him to do his rah-rah imitation of the university player is criminal negligence on the part of parents, and its damaging effect is likely to handicap the boy through life. Suitable athletic contests for growing boys should be limited to short rounds of boxing, sprints, swimming, baseball, tennis and jumping.

The individual with a heart valve deficiency, or a heart muscle lesion (myocarditis, fatty degeneration, etc.), or a narrowing of the coronary artery which supplies the heart muscle with blood, is handicapped with respect to ordinary mild activity exactly like the untrained or insufficiently trained athlete in a gruelling contest of endurance and effort.

It is a popular notion that anyone with any kind of heart trouble must avoid all exercise. This is wrong in most cases. Graduated exercise, under the supervision of the physician, is the best way to develop reserve power when the heart is crippled by disease. The physician must prescribe such therapeutic exercise to suit the individual requirements, just as the physician prescribes any medicine, diet or rest he considers best for the patient's present condition.

Young men who have had some years of athletic training commonly develop some enlargement of the heart. This is unavoidable in training for contests of endurance such as football and other college sports. While the boys continue their athletics the enlarged heart gives no trouble, but should they abruptly change to some sedentary occupation they are likely to suffer from palpitation, consciousness of the action of the heart or other such symptoms. The college athlete, after graduation, would therefore be wise to continue one form or another of daily exercise rather than to break off suddenly. His cardiac hypertrophy was developed gradually— let it abate in the same gradual way.

When valvular leakage develops as a result of endocarditis complicating some such illness as quinsy, scarlet fever or acute infectious arthritis, the natural course of the valvular disease is gradual enlargement of the heart. When the heart is thus enlarged or hypertrophied and its capacity to maintain efficient circulation is increased, physicians refer to the state as "compensation" or "good compensation." Such a heart pumps an adequate supply of oxygen to the cells, tissues and organs to enable them to carry on their functions normally—so long as the individual's ways of living and his activities remain within his limitations or do not make greater demands than his margin of reserve power can meet. So it seems that enlargement of the heart can be a blessing.

As already explained, there may be no symptoms or signs to show that anything is the matter at the time acute or chronic endocarditis develops, unless the physician keeps the possibility of such complication in mind and watches the patient closely. This is the main reason why the physician commonly prescribes REST IN BED in the acute or early stage of many illnesses, even though the patient may feel able to be up and about. The victim of endo- carditis (inflammation of heart lining) becomes aware that some- thing is wrong only after weeks or months, when the inflammatory exudate or "vegetations" resulting from the lodgement of the bac- teria in the heart lining membrane begin to interfere with perfect seating of the heart valve and there is leakage back through the damaged valve at each heart beat. Of course this happens only when the portion of lining membrane covering the valve is affected; endocarditis elsewhere in the heart does no permanent harm.

So you see, the individual with endocarditis may be serenely un- aware of his illness and experience manifestations of circulatory deficiency only weeks or months after the acute stage has passed.

Since the essential purpose of circulation is to supply oxygen to the body cells, the most emphatic symptom of any impairment, weakening or failure of circulation, is breathlessness or labored breathing, panting on slight exertion or in some instances constant dyspnea (difficult, labored breathing, panting, puffing or wheezing).

The condition of the individual with such circulatory or heart deficiency is comparable with the condition of a man running a marathon race. Naturally you begin to get a bit "winded" at the end of the first half mile or so, but if you're in normal health, you get "second wind" somewhere around the end of the first mile.

But here the similarity ceases. The individual with valvular deficiency or even just flabbiness of the heart muscle has only sufficient heart power to maintain circulation while he is at rest or during very moderate exertion. If he is subject to demand for greatly increased oxygen supply, as in sudden, violent or prolonged effort, he hasn't the necessary margin of reserve power in his heart to call into service, so he never quite gets "second wind." He must either refrain from making the effort at all or risk complete collapse.

REMEDIES FOR VALVULAR LEAKAGE   The most familiar sign of valvular leakage is a "murmur"—a humming, blowing or purring sound heard with the stethoscope in addition to the normal "loved-up, loved-up, loved-up" sound produced by the beating of the heart. A murmur may be heard in cases of simple anemia when there is no valvular lesion or leakage at all. On the other hand, in cases of valvular disease, with loss of compensation, exhaustion of the reserve power and dilatation of the heart, the murmur which has been present may cease for a time and return only with beginning recovery of compensation or reserve power. To the physician an audible murmur may have some diagnostic or prognostic significance. The layman, sick or well, half-informed or uninformed, had better not try to gauge its meaning.

The accent is on the "loved," or more phonetically the "lub," the first sound, in the young of heart, the normal, healthy person. This sound is produced by the simultaneous contraction of the muscle of the ventricular walls and the closing of the valves between auricles and ventricles. The second sound, "up" or more phonetically "dup," is produced by the closure of the aortic and pulmonary valves, after blood has been pumped into the great artery (aorta) or into the pulmonary artery.

In any condition where the arterial tension is increased the second heart sound, the "up" or "dup" may be accentuated. Increased arterial tension (high blood pressure) is generally a compensatory change in the beginning or the early stages of the trouble, a conservative change which is essential to maintain adequate circulation despite the handicap, abuse, strain or degeneration which is developing. For this reason it is usually unwise to attempt to reduce high blood pressure by drugs, diet, baths and the like without careful consideration of the effect such interference may have on the circulation.

What remedies are available for valvular leakage?

Aside from a more careful adherence to the rules of good hygiene which valvular leakage imposes on the patient for life, no particular treatment is necessary when the heart is hypertrophied, enlarged sufficiently to compensate for the leakage; that is, when it is evident that the heart pumps more blood than the normal volume at each beat to compensate for the amount of blood that leaks back through the damaged valve at each beat. It is only when compensation is lost and there is evidence that the organs and tissues are not receiving sufficient blood that treatment is essential.

The first and best remedy is REST. Perhaps a week or ten days in bed will suffice to restore compensation in some cases, at least enabling the overtaxed heart to recover a narrow margin of reserve power.

Perhaps the best form of exercise to try carefully after the heart has recovered a little reserve power is Belly Breathing. The muscular effort involved in this is slight and each inflation of the bellows helps to pull more blood back from the great veins toward the lungs.

Later in the course of treatment carefully graduated EXERCISE taken strictly as prescribed by the physician to suit the individual case may be of great value in promoting hypertrophy, enlargement or increased muscular development of the heart necessary to widen the margin of reserve power so that the patient may lead a reasonably active life.

In my judgment graduated exercise is a heart tonic second only to B-Nutron. It should be graduated like this:

First day do the belly breathing exercise morning and evening. Second day do the exercise and also get out of bed into armchair for a few minutes morning and evening.

Third day add a leisurely walk around the room morning and evening. Fourth day the same, plus a walk down the corridor and back, morning and evening.

Fifth day the same, plus a walk of a hundred yards morning and evening. Sixth day the same, plus a walk around the block morning and evening. And so on, day by day a little farther until you can enjoy a stroll of a mile or two morning and evening.

QUESTION OF ALTITUDE   Changing from a low or moderate to a high altitude is equivalent to increasing the work of the heart by taking more active or prolonged exercise. Whether such a change of residence is advisable in cases of valvular or other heart trouble of course depends on the compensation or reserve power, and this is a question each patient's own physician can best answer.

As a rule a person with heart or artery trouble feels no distress at altitudes up to 7000 feet. Some even believe they feel better at such altitudes. A few may worry about shortness of breath on exertion, but that is also the experience of many healthy persons for the first few days.

Traveling over passes 10,000 feet high gives little discomfort, but remaining overnight or all day at such altitudes should be avoided until there has been some acclimatization.

These rules apply to flying also.

Schott baths, which are saline baths highly charged with carbon dioxide, as employed at Nauheim and at Saratoga Springs and other health resorts or sanitariums in this country, are beneficial in the treatment of decompensation, whether in valvular disease, myocarditis or cardiovascular disease in general. Artificial Schott baths may be given at home but only if skilled nursing and the personal supervision of a physician are available. For those who can afford it, a stay in a sanitarium where such baths are administered is more satisfactory. The physiological effect of carbon dioxide on the vasomotor (sympathetic) nervous mechanism which controls the circulation is manifest in the general improvement which patients receiving the baths show from day to day.

HERE IS A REAL HEART TONIC   A tonic is a remedy which restores enfeebled function and promotes vigor and a sense of well being. Food, air, water, sleep, rest, heat, cold, light and security— for instance the newborn infant safe and warm in mother's arms— may be a tonic in special circumstances.

A stimulant is not a tonic. A whip stimulates a tired horse. An extra measure of oats and a brief rest keeps the horse in fine fettle.

In my opinion no drug or medicine is a heart tonic. As for digitalis, although I would take it in only one conceivable circumstance, many good physicians still believe it is of value in the treatment of heart disease in decompensation, dilatation and the congestive phase, and they seem pretty confident in the rationale of its use. But as I say, I would take it only if my doctor ordered me to take it or else. I don't know how long I'd be willing to go along, but I'd take it or else fire the doctor.

The real heart tonic I recommend can do no harm and may do considerable good not only for the heart and circulation but for the digestion and nerves as well. It is not medicine at all. It is my same old remedy, simply food; food which every child or adult needs to maintain good digestion and good circulation but which few children or adults get in adequate proportions because of our ultra-refined diet. It is vitamin B complex, an optimal, daily ration of it. For children a teaspoonful daily, for adults a tablespoonful daily of B-Nutron Syrup; or, if preferred, for children one B-Nutron tablet or for adults three tablets daily. The tablets are chocolate coated.

The syrup is a pleasant vehicle for digitalis, iron or other unpleasant medicine. If you take digitalis regularly as a heart "tonic" I earnestly recommend that you take it with or in a good daily ration of B-Nutron Syrup and gradually reduce the dose of digitalis— say cut it in half at intervals of a week—until you take none at all. Continue the B-Nutron long after you have stopped the digitalis. In the course of a few months you will realize how much good a real heart tonic can do.

And when you do begin to enjoy that sense of well-being, give a little more thought and study to the problem of restoring the staff of life, plain wheat, to your everyday diet, for wheat is the richest food source of vitamin B complex.

Chapter Twenty-two

THE HEART'S SPECIFIC
DISEASES AND CARE

"Had Heberden listened to my first lecture," said Dr. Osler in a lecture on angina pectoris forty years ago, "he could have remarked very justly: 'Well! they have not got much ahead since my day.' "

If Dr. Osler could read this little lesson on heart and arteries he might fairly comment, "O ho, so they're still theorizing concerning the nature and cause of angina pectoris, are they!"

William Heberden, the 18th century English physician and scholar, first described the disease known today as angina pectoris and in Heberden's day called *pectoris dolor*—pain in the breast, or breast pang, breast meaning the chest. Heberden himself used the name angina pectoris. Of the seizure he wrote, "The seat of it, and sense of strangling, and anxiety with which it is attended, may make it not improperly called angina pectoris." The word angina is derived from the Greek root meaning to choke. It has been applied at various stages of medical history to croup, quinsy and several other inflammatory affections of the throat and is today most commonly applied to the infection popularly known as trench mouth, which manifests itself rather by sores in the mouth than by any great throat trouble.

On opening the body of one who died suddenly of this disease, wrote Heberden, a very skillful anatomist could discover no fault in the heart, in the valves, in the arteries or neighboring veins, excepting some small rudiments of ossification in the aorta.

That's the difficulty. There is no apparent organic change to account for the attacks of angina pectoris. So we really have not got much ahead since Osler's day.

Theories we have a-plenty. Don't we always have a good theory to account for what we do not understand?

I always plump for the anoxia theory as the most plausible. This means oxygen deficiency in the heart muscle. Treatment based on this conception gives excellent results, both inhalations of oxygen or, better still, carboxygen, a mixture of oxygen with seven per cent carbon dioxide. Another technique is subcutaneous injection of nascent oxygen gas.

Every sufferer from angina pectoris should carry at all times a few tablets of nitroglycerin, otherwise called glonoin or glyceryl trinitrate, each tablet containing from 1/100th to 1/200th of a grain. Such a tablet, dissolved in the mouth, acts in two minutes. It is not a heart stimulant. It is a vasodilator, which means it causes relaxation or dilation of the affected arteries. Dilation of the coronary arteries which supply blood to the heart muscle brings more blood and more oxygen, to the muscle cells. Any adult may take such a dose of nitroglycerin without danger. Many angina patients take such a dose three or four times a day for weeks or months with benefit and without untoward effect of any kind.

If the law permits druggists in your community to sell nitroglycerin tablets without prescription, that's fine. If not, there's nothing I can do about it except suggest that you ask some physician to write a prescription for a dozen or perhaps twenty tablets.

Some physicians and some patients prefer milder one-grain tablets of sodium nitrite for emergency use—one grain of sodium nitrite is equivalent to about 1/100th grain of nitroglycerine, but less abrupt and more prolonged in action.

Since medicine converted from profession to business, some doctors have virtually discarded nitroglycerin and sodium nitrite in favor of expensive prescription nostrums which purport to give the desirable effects of nitroglycerin but without any undesirable effects. In my judgment the claims the nostrum manufacturers make for these more expensive medicines are specious. The average dose gives the same effect as half the average dose of nitroglycerin or sodium nitrate. Anyone taking nitroglycerin should have enough gumption to regulate his own dosage and also to be able to determine whether his supply of tablets has become inert through volatilization.

COFFEE IS GOOD FOR THE HEART Excessive daily indulgence in tea or coffee—the effects are virtually the same except that a cup of coffee is equivalent to approximately two or three cups of tea—produces nervousness, insomnia, digestive disturbances, weakened eyesight and morning headache.

But many valetudinarians deny themselves coffee because they take seriously the propaganda of certain commercial interests which implies that coffee drinking causes heart disease and/or high blood pressure.

If these poor people derive satisfaction from such self-denial there's no great harm in it. But unless the attending physician specifically prohibits the use of coffee, people with heart trouble, particularly coronary trouble, derive real benefit from one or two cups of coffee at breakfast and, if desired, another cup at dinner time. The happy effect of coffee in such moderation is to keep the coronary arteries dilated, open or relaxed so that they deliver the full supply of blood (oxygen) to the heart muscle.

CORONARY THROMBOSIS Coronary arteries, right and left, branch from the aorta just beyond the aorta heart valve and supply blood to the heart wall itself.

Thrombus is a medical term for blood clot, and the ending *osis* means disease. So coronary thrombosis, otherwise known as cardiac thrombosis, is formation of a blood clot in some part of the coronary artery, restricting or completely shutting off the supply of blood to the portion of the heart fed by that branch of the artery. The result of such occlusion of the artery is infarct, or mortification of the portion of heart wall deprived of oxygen.

All this may be pretty complicated to the layman, and it is as far as seems wise to go into the morbid details. I give this information to enlighten the reader regarding the significance of terms often used in the newspapers, for a general understanding of such terms is less frightening than misconception of what they mean.

The only safe and sane course for anyone who has or believes or fears he has any kind of heart disease is to go to a doctor, leave it to him to determine just what is the matter, then follow instructions.

NEVER MIND YOUR BLOOD PRESSURE In the "doctor's bible" Osler says that longevity is a vascular question. Vascular pertains to the blood vessels. Everyone has heard the old axiom that a man is as old as his arteries. According to that fatalistic view, how long you may expect to live depends on the quality of the material your immediate and remote ancestors have put into your arteries. I shall not be positive about this until I get along toward ninety, but up to now I am convinced that longevity depends rather on the way you live. It is a question of hygiene. Not merely knowledge of hygiene, though that is important, but the knowing how to apply the knowledge in your own life, despite the many obstacles and difficulties that conspire to defeat your best endeavors.

Cardiovascular disease or degeneration (CVD) is the general term physicians apply to the premature heart-artery deterioration or slow failure of circulation that accounts for physical or "nervous" breakdown at or before middle age. It is the conventional practice to attribute this incapacitation to "strenuous life," heavy business responsibilities, the high tension of American life and all that sort of hooey. There is about as much sense in that as in referring to booze as "stimulants;" no sober physician or pharmacologist today will attempt to argue that alcohol is a stimulant or in any way necessary or good for you; but plenty of tipplers and obscure "scientific authorities" subsidized by the alcoholic beverage interests will give you some such assurance if you are credulous enough to accept it.

Indulgence in alcoholic beverages, especially the vicious custom of drinking before dinner and the insidious habit of taking a drink as a pick-me-up or bracer when you feel tired or weary in the middle of the day's work or when the stomach is empty and perhaps the blood sugar low, is the actual factor of damage to the arteries, heart, liver and kidneys which people so readily ascribe to "nervous tension."

The relief such drinkers get from the pick-me-up is spurious—the alcohol merely dulls or benumbs consciousness of fatigue, depression or irritability. Taking any sort of food or food beverage such as an ice cream soda, milk, fruit juice, sweetened tea, cocoa, chocolate, fruit, candy, cake or nuts would bring more real refreshment and recovery, so far as restoration is possible without an interval or sleep. If one food or beverage is superior to another in refreshing effect, it is only because of the sugar it contains, any kind of sugar being most rapidly absorbed and utilized for combustion to provide immediate energy.

Oh, yes, blood pressure. Everybody is concerned about blood pressure. The average layman has a notion that blood pressure should be 100 plus your age or something like that. Notwithstanding this curious idea, blood pressure is of only minor or secondary significance. Your blood pressure is too high or too low in consequence of what ails you or of your way of living. You will never get anywhere if you are childish enough to believe that it has somehow gotten out of kilter when you weren't watching, so if you can only find some drug, diet or bath which will raise or lower it a few notches, as the case may be, your other complaints will vanish.

THROMBO-ANGITIS OBLITERANS   Young adults between the ages of 20 and 35 or 40 sometimes complain of pains in the foot, in the calf of the leg or in the toes, and particularly of a sense of numbness or coldness whenever the weather is unfavorable. Upon examination we see that one or both feet are markedly blanched, almost cadaveric in appearance, cold to the touch, and that neither the dorsalis pedis, the artery passing down front of instep, nor the posterior tibial artery, back of the calf and behind the inner prominence of ankle bone pulsates. When the foot becomes warm some color gradually returns.

That is the description of thrombo-angitis obliterans or Buerger's disease, quoted almost verbatim from the study published by Dr. Leo Buerger in American Journal of the Medical Sciences. Thrombo-angitis obliterans is otherwise known as presenile spontaneous gangrene, but since Buerger's work it is usually called Buerger's Disease.

Some patients complain of rheumatic pains in the leg, says Dr.

Buerger. Others are able to walk only short distances before the advent of paroxysmal shooting cramp-like pains in the calf of the leg forces them to stop short. Some of these cases show the typical symptoms of intermittent claudication. (There we go, using four-syllable words again! But intermittent claudication is merely a $50 term for spells of limping with intervals of freedom from limping.)

After months, in some cases even years, Dr. Buerger continues, trophic disturbances appear (trophic meaning pertaining to nutrition of the affected leg, foot or toes). It is at this stage that another rather unique symptom emerges—erythromelalgia, which means literally burning or throbbing pain in the limb with mottling or reddening of the skin. At first the skin around the toes and front of the foot becomes bright red when the foot hangs down. Later the skin shows first a small blister, then a hemorrhagic bleb and finally ulceration, perhaps on the tip of one toe. At this stage pain is intense and the patient finds little relief.

I hate to add that this is gangrene necrosis, death of the extremity involved, and amputation becomes imperative in such circumstances. As a pipe smoker I do not mind stressing that in most cases of Buerger's disease excessive smoking seems to be the main cause, and that it is cigarette smoking which seems to cause the most damage, perhaps merely because it is easier to chain-smoke than to keep lighting a pipe.

THE COURSE OF THROMBO-ANGITIS OBLITERANS (BUER-GER'S DISEASE)   At the earliest intimation of the onset of gangrene in a toe, says Dr. Saul S. Samuels, smoking must be prohibited. This is so important that we may expect marked relief from pain after the patient has stopped smoking for a few days. The New York authority clearly meant to say that such relief may be expected to come within a few days after the patient has stopped smoking period.

Most scientific investigators conclude that smoking tends to increase diastolic and systolic blood pressure. Some of them believe the effect on blood pressure is not due entirely to irritation of the vasomotor nerve centers but in part to some element in tobacco smoke which produces constriction or narrowing of the finest or terminal arterioles. Two such investigators, Maddock and Collier, scientifically measured the effects of cigarette smoking in young adult males with thrombo-angitis. When these young men smoked a few cigarettes they showed a consistent increase of blood pressure and pulse rate and a decrease in the skin temperature of fingers and toes. These effects were more marked if the subjects "inhaled" while smoking and if they smoked rapidly rather than just puffed or smoked slowly. The authors do not contend however that smoking is the sole cause of thrombo-angitis obliterans, for they say the occurrence of the disease in individuals who have never smoked precludes that opinion.

From all this I infer that any smoker who suffers from coldness or blanching of the toes or forward part of foot or feet had better beware. I further advise every smoker to give himself the benefit of moderation if the smoking is to be continued at all.

In the earlier stages of thrombo-angitis obliterans the victims generally consult a "foot" specialist and in my observation the charlatan usually makes a show of trying to cure the trouble with his special arch prop or manipulation for some structural displacement or derangement he discovers in the foot or feet.

Then, too, men in the early stages like to think their trouble is "rheumatism" and follow plausible diets or take whatever treatment for "rheumatism" happens to appeal to their credulity.

Human nature, I suppose. But while they are indulging in such antics, unfortunately they usually keep on smoking and realize only too late where they have gone wrong.

MANAGEMENT OF BUERGER'S DISEASE   The impression that amputation of a leg is to be expected in most cases of Buerger's disease is erroneous. It is even wrong to think that amputation is necessary in every instance in which gangrene does occur. As shown by Dr. Saul S. Samuels, gangrene is a self-limiting process and extreme conservatism in even severe forms of gangrene is usually rewarded with an intact extremity. Amputation is advisable only when the gangrene has destroyed so much tissue that a nonfunctioning foot would be the outcome. Pain is no indication for amputation.

The patient with Buerger's disease should never sit with foot hanging down, but always keep it horizontal or perhaps elevated a little above hip level.

Injection of about ten fluid ounces of five percent hypertonic solution of sodium chloride into the veins every alternate day is probably the best way to supply a sufficient amount of fluid to the tissues affected. Or the fluid may be administered by injection under the skin, or by means of a duodenal tube. Some physicians believe that Ringer's solution, which contains not only sodium chloride but also calcium chloride, potassium chloride and sodium bicarbonate, is preferable to plain salt solution. If I were the patient I believe I would too.

Dr. Buerger himself recommends this exercise:

"The affected limb is elevated, with the patient lying in bed, from 60 to 90 degrees above horizontal, being allowed to rest upon a support for from 30 seconds to three minutes, the period being the minimum time necessary to produce blanching.

"As soon as blanching is established, the patient allows the foot to hang down over the edge of the bed for from two to five minutes, until reactionary hyperemia or rubor (reddening) sets in, the total period of time being about one minute longer than that necessary to establish a good red color.

"The limb is then placed in the horizontal position for about three to five minutes, during which time an electric heating pad or a hot water bag is applied, care being taken to prevent occurrence of a burn.

"The placing of the limb in these three successive positions constitutes a cycle, the duration of which is usually from six to ten minutes. These cycles are repeated over a period of about one hour."

A daily half hour of medical diathermy, using a foot plate and cuff below knee or, if there is no pulsation in the popliteal artery, cuff above the knee, gives considerable relief from pain in some cases.

Of course, there is no reasonably safe pain-killer the patient can take frequently or habitually. It becomes a problem for the physician to select the medicine which may do the least possible harm when a pain-killer is necessary regularly.

Once blistering, blebs, ulceration or any kind of sore or fester develops, perhaps under the edge of a nail, it is vitally important that the care of the limb be supervised by the physician. The foot and leg should be given daily hot baths containing an antiseptic and deodorant such as chloramine in weak solution, say one-half teaspoonful in the quart of water.

VITAMIN E IS NOT A REMEDY FOR HEART TROUBLE   In 1950 and '51 queries concerning the remedial value of vitamin E for heart trouble were at a peak. In '52 and '53 popular interest in this wonderful new remedy steadily declined. Since then vitamin E has lost interest.

Among 260 reports on vitamin E published in scientific journals by physicians, veterinaries, nutrition investigators, chemists and other authorities, many dealt with its value in the treatment of muscular dystrophy, progressive muscular atrophy. However, not one substantiated the claim that vitamin E is of any special benefit in heart disease. Nutrition authorities believe that everyone needs a certain amount of vitamin E daily and that if the diet is deficient in it, such conditions as abortion, poor muscular development in infants and muscular dystrophy are likely to occur, but just how much a person requires has not yet been determined.

The best natural food source of vitamin E is plain wheat. The decrease of vitamin E in modern diets caused by the use of refined white flour makes it probable that the average diet is on the edge of deficiency.

TOBACCO HEART   In addition to the observations of Maddock and Collier mentioned earlier, it may be well again to quote Dr. Osler's *Practice of Medicine:* "There are three groups of cases of so-called tobacco heart: First, the irritable heart of smokers, seen particularly in young lads, in which the symptoms are palpitation, irregularity, and rapid action; secondly, heart pain of a sharp, shooting character, which may be very severe; and, thirdly, attacks of such severity that they deserve the name of angina."

Speaking as the owner of a large herd of pipes I can add that almost invariably these and other pathological effects do occur in tobacco hogs—smokers who indulge to excess.

A REMEDY FOR RESTLESS LEGS   A common complaint of mature adults with poor circulation is that their legs are restless when they try to relax and get to sleep nights. They can't find a position that is comfortable for any length of time. The remedy here is nitroglycerin, otherwise called trinitrin, glyceryl trinitrate and, formerly, glonin.

It is difficult, however, and in most places impossible to purchase nitroglycerin tablets without prescription—of course the prescription of your own physician. It may be that your physician or any physician you happen to know will give you a dozen nitroglycerin tablets, each containing 1/100th of a grain.

The rapid action of nitroglycerin, described in the chapter on *pectoris dolor,* more familiar as *angina pectoris,* may mislead the uninitiated to regard the medicine as too "powerful" and therefore too "dangerous." Be that as it may, many physicians and specialists advise patients subject to cardiovascular troubles to carry nitroglycerin tablets in pocket or purse and pop one in the mouth at any time distress occurs or even threatens. Sometimes physicians recommend that such persons take small doses of nitroglycerin or other vasodilator more or less regularly four or five times a day.

Habit? Conceivably such medicine may eventually give less relief when the body becomes used to or resistant to it, but if regular, frequent or occasional doses gave me relief or comfort I'd enjoy the relief or comfort without concern about habituation.

For the complaint of "restless legs"—and this does not mean cramp, pain or dull ache—it is advisable to take at first only one-half of a 1/100th-grain tablet of nitroglycerin—dissolve it in the mouth after you get into bed. Then just lie there repeating the Pater Noster in Latin or the Twenty-third Psalm in any language. In six of the former or four of the latter you will know whether the medicine is working or whether the tablets are inert. If it is working you will experience relief or perhaps flushing of your face or throbbing in your head for a few minutes. Then as you simmer down again the relief you sought will come.

Nitroglycerin is so volatile that tablets, even when kept in tightly stoppered vials, steadily lose strength. The only way to make sure a supply of the tablets is not inert is by taking one and waiting a few minutes for the characteristic reactions. If one or two tablets dissolved in the mouth have no effect within two or three minutes, throw the whole lot away and get some fresh ones.

To relieve restless legs at night take one nitroglycerin tablet after getting into bed and a second tablet at any time more than five minutes later.

POPULAR OBSESSIONS ABOUT THE HEART   Contrary to common belief:

Real heart disease only rarely causes sudden death.

Persons subject to valvular disease, myocarditis, or cardiovascular degeneration associated with arteriosclerosis are as likely to succumb at last to some illness like pneumonia as they are to die of "heart failure."

Most patients with heart disease discover the fact that the heart is affected only months or years after the beginning of the trouble, and then only incidentally in a life insurance examination or a "health survey" they are obliged to undergo. It will take many years of education to persuade any considerable proportion of people past 30 to spend their perfectly good cash for annual or periodic voluntary health examinations. That sort of prophylaxis can have no great appeal to the Yankee mind as long as the corner drugstore offers an infinite variety of quick relief for whatever the ailment.

When symptoms do occur during development of heart disease, they do not point to the heart. Rather they are in the form of slight breathlessness or short-windedness on exertion, slight cough, perhaps occasional swelling of ankles or feet toward evening, greater fatigue from ordinary activity and the inference that you are "run down from overwork" and need a vacation.

Palpitation, pains in the general region of the heart, a sensation as though the heart "skips beats" are frequent complaints in minor ailments but seldom indicative of heart disease.

Old time physicians with little or no scientific knowledge of the chemistry of nutrition conceived a theory, which survives in popular fancy. This theory holds that too much calcium in food or water might cause hardening of the arteries, gallstones, kidney stones and chronic arthritis. Neither physiologist, biological chemist, nutritionist nor medical authority holds that anyone ever absorbs more calcium from food, water or medicine than the body requires for health. We may take it as established that hard water of satisfactory taste is perfectly healthful for anyone to drink, and foods rich in calcium are as healthful for mature adults or for children as they are for infants.

THE NUTRITIONAL FACTOR OF CVD   If you suffer from cardiovascular disease you should be sure to get an adequate daily ration of calcium and vitamin D, from food and/or food supplement. Calcium is tonic to the heart muscle. It tends to keep the coronary and other arterioles relaxed and the blood pressure down.

No recognized medical authority, no pathologist, can show that "calcium deposits" or calcification in the coats or walls of arteries causes arteriosclerosis or hardening of the arteries. Actually such change in artery walls is a *consequence*, an advanced stage of sclerosis. Incidentally it is notable that the "experts" or "scientific authorities" who issue warnings of the "danger" that "too much calcium" and/or vitamin D may cause "calcium deposits" or calcification of arteries and joints, never say how much is "too much." I suspect most of them don't even know how much calcium and vitamin D we require daily to maintain VITE.

THE ABUSE OF ANALGESIC DRUGS   I cannot repeat too often that a large number of aniline or coal tar derivatives used in medicine for the relief of ache, pain or other unpleasant sensations are more or less injurious to the heart, the blood and the central nervous system. These drugs, under their own name or disguised in various popular nostrums, are used indiscriminately by people who are either uninformed or only vaguely aware of their possible dangers. In their naive way they assume that the government would not permit the sale of a nostrum containing a dangerous quantity of a dangerous drug, especially when the nostrum masquerades under a fancy name which gives no indication that acetanilid or phenacetin is its chief ingredient.

The aniline or coal tar derivatives to which I refer and which

I also discuss in the chapter on aspirin are acetanilid, otherwise called phenylacetamide; phenacetin, otherwise called acetphenetidin; aminopyrone, otherwise called pyramidon and amidopyrine; aspirin, otherwise called acetylysalicylic acid; phenobarbital, otherwise called luminal, veronal, barbiturate or sodium amytal.

A great many nostrums enjoying unrestricted sale to the public are virtually mixtures of one or another of these analgesics with ingredients which are practically inert or of secondary importance —ingredients used merely to afford an excuse for giving the nostrum a misleading or deceptive name calculated to make the unwary buyer think it is mainly quinine or mainly bromide, since these are comparatively harmless medicines.

According to coroners' verdicts there have been numerous deaths from acetanilid poisoning due to a nostrum available as freely as a fountain drink—one to which people are urged to resort for such trifling discomfort as "brain fag" or "shopper's fatigue." This is a type of popular medicine which is a scandal to our national intelligence and honesty.

To take drugs indiscriminately in the early stage of an illness which, for all you or even your doctor knows, may be pneumonia, is a reckless way to gamble with life. Each dose destroys a few more blood corpuscles, interferes with the oxygen-carrying function of the hemoglobin in the blood and increases the anoxia or oxygen deficit in the body cells, particularly in the heart muscle. Anoxia is the lethal feature in heart disease.

In some circumstances, of course, relief of pain or other distress by one or another coal tar analgesic is rational, justifiable and good treatment. But in any case it is a question wisely put to the judgment of your physician.

Our federal government has piddled with the vital question of dangerous or habit-forming drugs for many years, beginning with the highly questionable "Pure Food and Drugs Act of June 30, 1906" which was the most unblushing betrayal of the welfare and safety of the people that the federal government ever perpetrated. They bowed down to the nostrum makers—and left the dumb public to hold the bag. This same spirit animates our federal government's present food and drugs bureau. Although that bureau makes regulations which purport to compel the medicine manufacturer to give a name to his product that will indicate its chief ingredient, or to forbid him from giving it a name which conveys the suggestion that some insignificant ingredient is the chief one, this whole regulation doesn't actually make the big nostrum interests behave but merely discourages some little fellows from competing with the interests that have plenty of loose funds to hand out to their lobbies. How else do the big nostrum interests continue selling the Yankee public all their bromo-compounds and quinine-compounds which are actually nothing but disguised acetanilid or phenacetin?

Not only for safety but for the most efficient action of medicine, it is an excellent rule to lie down for an hour at least whenever you take any analgesic drug, whether aspirin, antipyrin, aminopyrin or one of the barbiturates. In this way you will get the desired deadening of sensation of pain or distress with a smaller dose of the dope and correspondingly less damage to heart, central nervous system and blood.

CATCH YOUR HEART FAILURE EARLY   Despite all efforts to convince "well" people of the wisdom and economy of the practice of undergoing a periodic voluntary health examination once a year, especially after the age of 30, the great majority still put off seeing a doctor until failing health and strength make it evident they can no longer carry on. Oddly enough many who should have medical examination and advice, but don't, give as the main reason the prohibitive cost which they can't afford, yet in a year or two of piddling they spend perhaps many times what proper medical advice would have cost in the first place and spend it for worthless nostrums which purport to be good for this and that complaint. As long as people generally elect to stumble along blindly rather than face their health status and limitations, it is unlikely that any material progress can be made toward the control of cardiovascular disease by modern preventive medicine. Vital statistics show that although there has been a steady decline in the prevalence of most life-destroying disease in the past three decades, cancer and cardiovascular disease not only continue as prevalent as ever but seem to be actually on the increase. This increase among the people of the United States may in fact be only apparent, since a far greater proportion of cases of cancer and of cardiovascular disease are properly diagnosed today thanks to more accurate and universal use of precise diagnostic methods.

Let us not be cynical about this. There is a great deal more for the man or woman past 30 to gain from an annual medical examination than a chance to become another mortality statistic. I am a therapeutic nihilist—highly skeptical of the value of medicines applied as remedies or cure. But I do believe thoroughly in preventive medicine, correct hygienic and optimal nutrition. I sincerely believe that, if taken in time, both cancer and cardiovascular disease may be cured. I am convinced they are cured in a good many cases by timely correction of bad hygiene, faulty nutrition, neglected sources of irritation or focal infection.

Still speaking of cardiovascular degeneration and still mindful that there are no definite symptoms by which either the patient or the physician can recognize any form of artery or heart disease, we mention here some of the symptoms or complaints which should warn any intelligent adult of the need of a careful physical or health examination:

If you become easily fatigued if you maintain mental effort, as in reading or writing for a short time.

If you become forgetful of details of your work or of recent events.

If you require longer hours of rest and you do not recuperate as quickly with rest as you formerly did.

If you can't run half a mile or even a few blocks at any pace—you get winded too easily.

If you have digestive difficulties unknown in earlier years, especially a sense of fullness or bloating and of "gas."

If you are becoming somewhat corpulent, flabby, disinclined to indulge in exercise or effort you formerly enjoyed.

If your skin has grown sallow, harsh and dry; your eyes dull and often congested.

If your spirits are not so cheerful as they were when you were in your prime.

CORRECTIVE PROTECTIVE DIET

Breakfast:

	Calories
Glass of orange juice	100
Two eggs	166
Fresh fruit	80
Glass of milk	160

Luncheon:

One-third head of lettuce	16
Tablespoonful of oil	93
Two fresh vegetables	80
One pat of butter	95
Two glasses of milk	332
Fresh fruit	80

Dinner:

Meat	190
One-third head of lettuce	16
Tablespoonful of oil	93
Two fresh vegetables	80
One pat of butter	95
One glass of milk	160
Fresh fruit	80
Cheese	90
Handful of nuts	140

As listed the diet yields approximately 2200 calories, which is barely a maintenance ration for an adult at rest. A sedentary adult who takes little exercise requires 2500 to 2800 calories. One who gets an adequate amount of daily exercise, in work, play or downright treadmill calisthenics, needs 3300 or more calories. The regimen outlined is therefore a reduction diet for any adult not confined to bed or chair.

It not only gives an alkaline ash, which opposes acidosis, but it contains an ample quantity of the essential mineral elements, such as calcium and phosphorus. I believe this diet is adapted for keeping and building sound teeth, and one following such a regimen has no more need for brushing the teeth than has a savage from deepest Africa.

The chief feature of the diet, however, is the proportion of "protective foods" it contains. Every item in it, except lean meat and salad oil, is rich in vitamins, and we know now that it is the vitamin deficiency of our modern refined foods that accounts for the nutritional troubles we have gropingly ascribed to overeating, poorly balanced diet, wrong combinations, insufficient mastication, irregular meats, faulty cooking, lack of mineral salts, insufficient roughage and lack of iron. The diet admirably covers the essentials— fresh dairy products, fresh fruit and vegetables, especially green leafy vegetables. Whether you can or do stick to the regimen or not, listing it will at least help you to remember the great value of these foods in everybody's diet.

ACIDOSIS   My own opinion is that one should not care whether a given food, meal or menu gives an acid or an alkaline ash, as an ordinary working rule. Perhaps the ill effects that have been ascribed to predominance of acid-ash items in the diet are really due to the coincidence that such a diet is deficient in vitamins. Thus bread, potatoes, tea, sugar, cake, pie, candy, ice cream, beans, jam, jelly, marmalade, cocoa, coffee, bacon and most so-called breakfast cakes or cereals, are all non-protective foods poor in vitamins.

Please understand clearly, I do not imagine any of these suggestions will cure anything. I offer them in the sincere belief that, if adopted by adults in the incipient stage of C.V.D. they may help to reverse or at least retard the degeneration process and restore or prolong the physical and mental efficiency of youth. And I can give assurance, based on extensive experience, that the remedial and hygienic measures I suggest can do no one harm.

In conclusion may I remind you that if and when you wish to do so, I'll be delighted to receive from you a brief report of your success. Such a note or message from a reader who has tried my medicine and found it beneficial is, you know, very good medicine for me.

Chapter Twenty-three

TONICS, MIRACLE DRUGS AND PLACEBOS

In horse and buggy days in Penn Yan on Lake Keuka, most beautiful of the Finger Lakes of Western New York, tonics were an important part of a doctor's stock in trade. People were a little leery of the doctor who wrote prescriptions. They felt that for their 50¢—equivalent to $5.00 today—the doctor ought to supply the medicine, and competition compelled him to do so.

This wasn't a serious problem when you made a house call. You merely put a spoonful of medicine in a glass of water and ordered mother or Aunt Jo to administer a teaspoon every hour. The cost of the medicine was perhaps a penny and the fee for the visit a dollar—if you could collect.

But patients who came to the office would be pretty upset if you charged more than 50¢, so that enough medicine to keep a patient going for a week might set you back a nickel. I cudgeled my brains to find a way to evade this ten percent tax on office practice, but in vain. Then one day an elder colleague told me not only how to evade the tax but also how to make a neat profit on the transaction. In ten years he had been very successful financially, built himself a fine new home, invested in mortgages on farm land and acquired a substantial share of stock in the bank. It was quite simple. Each patient received not only the usual free medicine but also an extra envelope or box of tablets for the blood, for the nerves, for the digestion—and that would be 25¢ extra. Thus the doctor made a clear profit of fifteen or twenty cents in addition to the 50¢ fee for office consultation. Listening to him describing the bonanza, I was delighted. I went home and put it into effect. But it didn't work well at all. I found, dammit, that I just couldn't charge poor people a quarter for two cents' worth of medicine when I knew they didn't need it.

Later, however, I did develop a good sideline—a tonic containing iron, quinine and one other ingredient I'd rather not mention. It was very bitter—that was the way a really good tonic had to taste—so bitter that it brought 50¢ per four-ounce bottle. Steady customers returned again and again or sent messengers for a refill.

Of course, it is conceivable that the medicine may have done good in some cases, but my face feels red even now when I think of the quantity of tonic I dispensed in my four years in Penn Yan merely to keep patients from changing doctors. Naturally the other doctors played the same game to keep *their* patients from running to the new doctor for some of *his* tonic.

A tonic, you understand, is a remedy which restores enfeebled function. It is not necessarily medicinal. One of the best tonics for a sedentary person, a professional or white collar worker is a two mile walk three times a day—once in the morning on the way to work, once around town at lunchtime, and finally a brisk walk home at night. The equivalent in any other kind of moderate general exercise will do almost as well.

As a therapeutic skeptic, I question whether any medicine may be considered a tonic. Many poor souls, for instance, have been persuaded to believe that a daily dose of digitalis was indispensable to them because of their "weak hearts." Some of them later discovered that not only could they do without digitalis and remain alive, but also that they regained a good deal of their former wellbeing by switching to the good old Brady heart tonic, which is nutritional, not medicinal. One or two teaspoonfuls daily of B-Nutron syrup or one or two B-Nutron tablets, virtually the same formula, is a *real* heart tonic, for it actually does improve the tone and function of involuntary muscle, such as the muscle coat of stomach and intestine and the muscle of heart and artery wall.

Digitalis (foxglove) was introduced to medicine by Dr. William

Withering in 1775 not as a heart stimulant or tonic but as a remedy for dropsy. Withering learned about it from an old woman in Shropshire. Today physicians seldom use it for dropsy or as a diuretic, which it is, but dote on it as a remedy for heart trouble.

"Therapeutically," says a modern textbook, "digitalis enables the damaged heart to do more work with the same expenditure of energy." If this makes sense I'll just go quietly, constable . . .

It is remarkable how satisfied people used to be when the doctor listened ten or 20 cents' worth to their complaints and then put his fingertips together and opined, "Well, what you need is a good blood tonic—" or tonic for the heart or for the nerves. The patients cheerfully accepted a bottle in lieu of a diagnosis.

And speaking of tonics, I am reminded of a nostrum that achieved great popularity among the intelligentsia about the time we said a tearful goodbye to Topsy the Beautiful Sorrel—a horse we've never forgotten since she coincided with the first three years of our marriage and the birth of Lalla Rookh.

The nostrum to which I refer wasn't touted as a tonic—there were too many of these cluttering druggists' shelves. It was "nerve food"—if you are an old timer you will remember how popular "neurasthenia", "nervous exhaustion" and "nervous breakdown" once were among the intelligentsia and how fashionable it was for the $500 snobs to go to the sanitarium for still more rest and relaxation when everybody at home was fed up.

Lawyers, college professors, clergymen, business executives, musicians, salesmen and others who lived without doing any honest work or getting any exercise wrote the finest testimonials for the stuff—or at least the vendor told the public so. After all, these people had more delicate or vulnerable "nerves" than lowbrows like you and me and they needed something more than ordinary victuals to maintain or restore nerve energy, whatever that may be. Myself, I never quite got the hang of it, for I didn't loaf four years in college between high school and medical school. All I learned in physiology, pathology, hygiene, prophylaxis and therapeutics was that energy is energy, whether expended in work or in play. I learned that a student expends a great deal more energy walking to and from college than he does taking an examination in mathematics or chemistry. And in physiology I learned that nerves, like telephone or telegraph wires, merely convey messages and use no energy at all. So it is pretty silly to yak about "nervous exhaustion," "weak nerves," "nervous prostration," "neurasthenia" or "nervous breakdown."

Samuel Hopkins Adams described the "nerve food" as *glorified cottage cheese,* and not long afterward it disappeared from the market. In retrospect it would seem that this "nerve food" had some virtue, for it contained nearly as much calcium and phosphorus as milk and egg yolk—foods which were spoon-fed to neurasthenics on a sojourn at the sanitarium.

The old timers, knowing only a little about chemistry and nothing about nutrition, imagined phosphorus was the important element and calcium unimportant or even harmful. So for a time persons with weak, delicate or bad "nerves" were plied with phosphates of this or that, syrup of hypophosphites, elixir of glycerophosphates and so on, although there is no evidence that in exhaustion states the nerve tissues lack phosphorus. Today most of these phosphorus-compounds have been discarded from the Pharmacopoeia.

In the days when the quacks and patent medicine people thrived on that great advertising gimmick, the free almanac, prospective customers spent the long winter evenings trying on for size the symptoms of "impure blood," "liver complaint," "catarrh," "female weakness" and what not. In one or another almanac they generally found symptoms to fit their case and purchased at least one bottle of the medicine extolled there. The nostrum vendors made it easy for customers to select the right medicine by calling their medicines Carter's Little *Liver* Pills, Doan's *Kidney* Pills, or Mayr's Wonderful *Stomach* Remedy—until the egregious Dr. Wiley came along and shamed Uncle Sam into a bit of house cleaning. After that Carter's Liver Pills became just Carter's Pills, Doan's Kidney Pills became just Doan's Pills, etc., and the customers had to select their medicine almost at random.

Mayr's Wonderful Stomach Remedy, advertised as a "positive and permanent cure for all stomach and intestinal ailments . . . appendicitis and gallstones," consisted of a large dose of olive, peanut or cottonseed oil followed by a saline cathartic. This combination normally produced soapy lumps in the intestine—pea size or chestnut size lumps which the victim persisted in believing were gallstones. The poor goofs used to bring these to me on a shingle when I practiced in Penn Yan, and it was impossible to convince them the lumps were merely soap.

I later knew Mayr in California—he was one of my bowling cronies—after he retired from the drug business in Chicago. He retired with a million or two, which by the way, he parlayed into a multimillion fortune in real estate investments.

George was a cigar smoker. He apparently enjoyed his smoking. I never could bring myself to ask how he could squander money for fancy cigars when it might do so much good in the world. You have to have respect for forty million dollars.

George saw how much I enjoyed my pipe. One day he asked me what kind of tobacco I smoked. I told him. "And how much does it cost?" It cost about $2.40 a pound at the time. George thought that was pretty steep. Next time I saw him he carried a little sack containing a 5-cent corncob pipe and a small pack of what purported to be tobacco, which set him back something like nine cents. He made an earnest effort to enoy the pipe, but, good grief, how could he?

Before he turned up his toes George was confined to his home for a few years. The home was high on a hill overlooking Beverly Hills. There were half a dozen bathrooms. When a maid, bent on keeping the place neat, collected odds and ends of used soap and placed fresh cakes in the bathrooms, Old George would make a tour of the house with the aid of his nurse and order the erring maid to replace the old bits of soap and put the new soap back in the store room until he called for it.

If we were passing the hat to give an unfortunate bowler some little token of our affection George would have no part of it.

And yet one of our three greens—we have the finest bowling greens in the country—which cost about $16,000, perhaps two or three times as much as bowling greens usually cost, is the gift of Mr. and Mrs. George H. Mayr. And when the man departed he left a fund, to be administered by a board of trustees, which gives financial assistance to deserving young people who want to go to college but lack the necessary means.

The moral of this story is, I suppose, that the fortunes made out of the public's bad health do, on occasion, revert to serve the public good. But this is a round-about way of going about it, to say the least.

HOPE FOR A MIRACLE   And speaking of morality, I would like to comment on something in the more recent past, the congressional inquiry into the outrageously high cost of proprietary drugs prescribed by physicians—or as I prefer to call them, the merchants of medicine. For a week or two people were scandalized by the facts as they appeared in the press. But the scandal soon died down and the customers, having accepted the fact that medical research is extremely expensive, resumed paying through the nose for the same fancy drugs. Obviously they were convinced that the trick specialists and the clinic men can do no wrong, otherwise they would all have by now gone back to "ordinary" doctors.

While the scandal was still the subject of timid comment in the magazines, a brand new nostrum was introduced in an eight-page spiel printed on de luxe special paper in the *Journal of the American Medical Association*. This nostrum bears a trade name printed in large letters, one easy for the doctor to memorize and write into their prescriptions. It also carries the generic name of the drug, but in unobtrusive small letters.

For what ailment will the specialists prescribe this medicine of great price? The ad spells it all out for them, covering a wide field in a single paragraph: "Indications: May be used for patients with hypercholesterolemia" (more than the average or usual amount of cholesterol in the blood) "and conditions thought to be associated with elevated cholesterol levels, including coronary artery disease (angina pectoris) and postmyocardial infarction and generalized atherosclerosis."

The medical dictionaries spell that first long word *hypercholesteremia*—but after all the firm introducing the nostrum had eight pages to fill!

As for "postmyocardial infarction" (which is defined as necrosis or death of a limited area of heart wall resulting from obstruction of a branch of the coronary artery which supplies blood to the heart muscle—obstruction by thrombus, that is, clot, as in coronary

thrombosis, or obstruction by embolus, such as air, fat or a frag-
ment of blood clot lodging in an arteriole)—when this happens,
it seems to me, prescribing medicine or diet to lower the level of
cholesterol in blood or tissues is exactly as effective as rushing out
to close the barn door after the horse has been stolen.

The term "atherosclerosis" is altogether nonsensical, and use of
it by a medical writer betrays ignorance of pathology. *Athero*
means softening and *sclero* means hardening. Come, now, ad boys,
you can't have it both ways. Either the artery or other tissue is
softened or else it is hardened. "Atherosclerosis" is strictly for the
birds—the poll-parrots and the ninnyhammers.

I had rather not ask a pharmacist what the new nostrum will
cost the retail customer but I can almost hear the gasp as he staggers
back under the impact of the pharmacist's price—the dose is one
250 mg.—approximately four grains—pearly gray capsule daily,
and the medicine is supplied in bottles of 30 capsules.

In view of the fact that this magic drug "may be used" for
patients who have "conditions THOUGHT to be associated with
elevated cholesterol levels," it seems to me that it can only help
those who dispense it. Even if we *knew* cholesterol to be the cause
of any of the conditions "thought to be associated" with elevated
cholesterol levels in the blood, it is only reasonable to expect that
it would take years and years of diet and medication to reverse
the process and get the cholesterol "deposits" out of the arteries
or other tissues. You would have to be an incurable optimist, and
completely ignorant of physiology, pathology and nutrition besides,
to hope for a miracle like that.

PLACEBOS   A placebo is a medicine or preparation, especially
an inactive one, given merely to satisfy a patient; an indifferent
substance, in the form of a medicine, given for the moral or sug-
gestive effect; or it may be a method of treatment that has no
remedial value but appeals to the patient's imagination. Even a
potent drug may serve as a placebo—for instance, the wee spot
of digitalis the valetudinarian must have every day to keep the
ticker going.

In *The New Yorker* Oct. 15, 1960, Berton Roueché cites various
medical journal reports on extraordinary benefits gained from the

use of placebos. For a fair and impartial evaluation of the remedial or curative effect of a new drug supposedly superior to drugs in current use, the investigator assigns arbitrary numbers to a group of persons with the disease or ailment in question, the numbers running from one to forty. Patients with odd numbers receive the medicine. Patients with even numbers receive only a placebo— something that looks like and perhaps even tastes like the real medicine. The record of the progress of the two groups after days or weeks of medication is illuminating. The odd number patients report virtually the same amount of relief from pain, stiffness and other symptoms as the even numbered group! It is only fair to mention here that in any case "the rheumatiz" (since I don't know what "arthritis" is) has good and bad days, periods when the victim is fairly comfortable and others when the stiffness, ache or pain is more pronounced.

In 1937 Dr. Harry Gold and his associates reported in the *American Heart Journal* that a placebo in many cases relieved the pain of angina pectoris as well as the conventional analgesic theobromine and aminophylline. Again in 1950 Gold and another group of associates found that a placebo relieved the pain of angina pectoris in as many cases—about one-third of all—as the drug Khellinine, derived from bishop's-weed, which was then being exploited as the best bet for that purpose.

The apparent effectiveness of placebos in these and other circumstances is not to be taken as evidence of deception or malingering. Rather it testifies to the power of suggestion.

Tranquilizers appear to be the most popular placebos at present —popular among people who are likely to become barbiturate addicts. The merchants of medicine are prescribing tranquilizers indiscriminately as placebos—medicine for complaints which the doctor doesn't understand. Newly rich, overprivileged women carry tranquilizers in their handbags and offer them to bridge party guests who are tired or worried. Tranquilizers enable such idle, useless women, to whom doing their own housework would be unthinkable, to evade conscientious scruples about their dreary, parasitic existence.

Doctors do not learn such therapeutics in medical school, in hospital, in textbooks or in postgraduate studies. They learn it from detail men—the traveling salesmen employed by pharmaceutical manufacturers—and from the full page or multi-page, elaborately colored ads of prescription nostrums in the medical journals. Of course they also learn to prescribe each nostrum by its proprietary or trade name, not by its generic or chemical name. This trick keeps the drug strictly a prescription item and makes it cost maybe three or four times what it would if you bought it under its generic name. This is very much the story of aspirin, once the patented proprietary or trade name for acetyl-salicylic acid. When the patent ran out and the manufacture and sale of aspirin was no longer restricted, anybody could make and sell it. The result is that today aspirin is aspirin no matter whether you pay the maximum or minimum price for it.

Hat in hand, bowing and scraping, a lowly family doctor recently wrote in to the AMA to inquire whether it was ethical for a general practitioner to dispense medicines to patients. To my astonishment the self-appointed arbiters of professional conduct assured the little man that it might be permissible under some circumstances. But they refrained from commending the doctor for thus protecting his patients from being exploited.

A revealing commentary on the extent to which medicine has been converted from a profession to a business in recent years was the leading article in the *Journal of the American Medical Association,* signed by a San Francisco practitioner, advising the young doctor who wants to succeed to go as heavily in debt as is necessary to enable him to drive the finest car and dress his wife in mink. These are the symbols the public recognizes . . .

There was a time when I co-operated with and had the cordial cooperation of the American Medical Association. But we fell out, or rather the Great Pooh-Bah and I fell out, when I protested against the high cost of insulin and the machinations by which the Association, then cringing under the heel of the dictator and flouting its own Code of Medical Ethics, approved the insulin patent and monopoly.

Instead of giving patients tranquilizers as placebos a physician can do no harm and may do much good by giving them something to combat or correct nutritional deficiency. Certainly most persons with minor complaints suffer from such deficiency. This is almost inevitable if more than half of the individual's daily calories come from refined white flour and refined white sugar. But here I go, riding my favorite hobby horse again.

Chapter Twenty-four

HOME'S THE PLACE TO HAVE A BABY

A college student in a small town in California received nation-wide newspaper publicity when he chained himself to his wife and so made it impossible for the hospital people to exclude him from the delivery room when their baby was being born. Perhaps this would solve the problem for other couples who want to share the miracle but find the hospital and even the doctor unalterably opposed to any such plan. While I admired and applauded the young man's courage I couldn't help chuckling at the remark the newspaper report ascribed to a doctor: "It just isn't sterile!"

The pretense of keeping the delivery room germ-free is absurd. Presence of the patient's husband is no more dangerous than the casual coming and going of nurses, interns, doctors or visiting firemen. I have yet to find hospital "rules and regulations" excluding from the delivery room doctors or nurses who are attending or have lately attended infectious or contagious illness—the "rules" leave that to the doctor's or nurse's conscience—which is not always aseptic.

Prospective parents who study *together* what all good husbands and wives should know about pregnancy, prenatal hygiene, childbirth and care of the baby obviously have dignity and self-respect to begin with. If there were more young couples of their intelligence level the star chamber delivery room would soon be converted to proper use.

Just what material is available for prospective parents to study?

Dozens of books, pamphlets and publications from federal and state government departments. To begin with there's a primer you can carry in your pocket or pocketbook, titled *Preparing for Maternity*. For a copy of this send 35¢ and a stamped envelope bearing your address to Dr. William Brady, 265 El Camino, Beverly Hills, California. For the 50-page *Brady Baby Book,* also pocket size, send another 35¢ and stamped self addressed envelope.

Maternity, a guide to prospective motherhood, is a fine book for expectant parents to study together. Without being insistent about it, the author, Frederick W. Goodrich, Jr., M.D., describes the advantages of natural childbirth and rooming-in. Published by Prentice-Hall, Inc., $1.75. Dr. Goodrich's other book, *Natural Childbirth,* a manual for expectant parents (Prentice-Hall, Inc., $3.50), is instructive to expectant parents, nurses and physicians. The author makes the point that study of the book will facilitate delivery whether the patient chooses natural childbirth or not.

Childbirth Without Fear is Dr. Grantly Dick Read's famous book about natural childbirth, published by Harper, and probably available in your public library. Whether prospective parents are sold on natural childbirth or not, reading Dr. Read's book will make them better parents.

The Modern Guide for Expectant Mothers, by Dr. Charles R. A. Gilbert (Hawthorn Books, Inc., Englewood Cliffs, N.J. $3.95) answers many questions which brides, wives and mothers sometimes hesitate to ask. Answers comply with the tenets of the Catholic church. It is the most informative book of its kind that has come to my notice in years.

The population of the infants' ward in the County Hospital in Buffalo, where I interned 20 months before beginning practice, was usually from 20 to 25, all of them the offspring of illegitimate parents. In most instances the mothers had been delivered in the hospital and discharged, leaving their babies for adoption. The babies were kept in the hospital, receiving the finest possible care for two years. Then, if not selected for adoption, then were transferred to an orphanage.

It was always a pleasure to make rounds in the babies' ward and see the nurses bathing, feeding, dressing and cuddling the little waifs. But the pleasant picture recalled an ugly one, that of the babies' own mothers so humanly, so unanimalistically deserting their young. And that in turn conjured up the still uglier picture of the father deserting both mother and child, yet retaining his standing in the community.

There was no monkey cage in the County Hospital to contain the anxious husbands, no corridor for them to pace. In fact there were no prospective fathers for the nurses to tranquilize.

Of course there was no plate glass show window nursery for the newborn, either and hence no spreading of infection from one infant to the other, as happens in many snooty lying-in institutions today. Each infant had his own crib, at least ten feet distant from the next infant. So there never was an epidemic of fatal infantile diarrhea, for instance, and that's one of the hazards of childbirth in some of the most pretentious hospitals today.

We didn't have what is now called "rooming-in" when I was an intern in the County Hospital, but the method of guarding the babies against infection was a good deal better than crowding them together in the glassed-in show window.

In a letter to the Editor of the San Francisco Chronicle, referring to the young man who padlocked himself to his wife, a lady said: "We felt from our own experience at the birth of our first child in Washington, D.C. that my husband's presence was a strong support to me and that it caused an unbreakable confirmation of our marriage union for us to share this miracle . . ." The editor's comment flabbergasted me: "Husbands and wives who wish to share this experience may not do so in California. It is prohibited here under a law enacted in 1946."

Then I received a letter from a Chicago man who asked how to surmount the regulation of the Illinois Department of Public Health which states: "No lay visitor, including relatives, shall be permitted in delivery rooms or nurseries."

I'm sure, cocksure if you please, that there's no such law in California or regulation in Illinois. If there is it is more honored in the breach than the observance.

Many readers have told me that when they engaged their obstetrician it was with the understanding that the expectant father would remain with his wife during the birth of the baby. Then when the time came the doctor would be so sorry—it was against the hospital's rules and regulations. People who haven't a home fit to have a baby in are not only timid souls but apparently stupid as well. At any rate the doctor hopes they are stupid when he plays that trick on them.

It is frightening to contemplate the great number of young married people who are prospective parents but still uneducated, unfit and too often unwilling to assume parental responsibility on their own. This character deficiency explains why such people go to a hospital to have a baby—it's a convenient way to evade responsibility.

These untutored prospective parents generally have not grown up. In high school they have been taught nothing at all about human embryology, prenatal hygiene, childbirth and infant care. Their own foolish parents and incompetent teachers have encouraged them to regard such subjects as not proper for innocent minds. Many queries pertaining to these subjects are shocking— shocking because they show deplorable ignorance and misinformation.

I admire and applaud a young Indiana couple who wanted to be together when their baby came. First they canvassed the physicians of their community and found none who would attend confinement unless the patient went to a hospital. In the face of such a situation most Americans would have given up and agreed to conform. But not this couple. They were determined to share the miracle of the birth of their baby, as human beings should. The expectant father was 18 or 19, a gas station attendant. The expectant mother was 17, and this was their first baby.

They might have called a licensed midwife, but they didn't. They just read all the pamphlets and books they could find. There are a good many books about childbirth available in bookstores and public libraries, and pamphlets obtainable from the state or provincial health department.

Thus when the time came the young woman bathed, put on a freshly washed and ironed nightgown and got into her sterile bed, made up with freshly laundered and ironed bed linen. And the young man scrubbed up, donned his freshly laundered gown and delivered his wife of an 8-pound baby.

These young people probably have a higher I.Q. and obviously far more gumption than the general run of prospective parents. When the doctors in their community tried to intimidate them, these young people did not panic. They did not throw themselves on the mercy of a hospital. They wanted to have their baby at home, the best place to have a baby, and they wanted to be together, not separated by hospital rules and regulations.

From what readers tell me about the baby business, it appears to be the practice not only in Indiana but throughout the country for doctors to refuse to attend childbirth at home. In effect this makes a federal case, so to speak, of every childbirth, and that's the way people with no gumption like it. A case in point is one pampered young woman who refused to listen to any discussion of natural childbirth, saying that when her time case she wanted to be rushed to the hospital, put under anesthesia and not wake up until it was all over.

In *Training for Childbirth: A Program of Natural Childbirth With Rooming-In,* by Herbert Thoms, M.D., (McGraw-Hill Book Company, Inc., New York, 1950, $3), the author says that support of the patient during labor is provided by the physician, the nurse, other attendants and the *patient's husband,* so that she retains confidence in her ability to see this physiological challenge through to a successful conclusion.

Jan Sterling, the movie actress, had her baby *at home* by natural childbirth, got up forty minutes later and walked about the room, combed her hair and put on some make-up. "The one thing that stands out in my mind," she said, "is that the actual birth is not painful at all. You just get the wonderful feeling that you have accomplished something important." She said she will do it the same way if she has another baby.

Approximately 85 per cent of babies born in the Santa Fe area served by the Catholic Maternity institute there are born at home by natural childbirth, attended by certified nurse midwives. "We don't call it 'natural childbirth'," said Sister Theophane. "We call it normal Christian childbirth."

"Four days ago," wrote a Massachusetts reader, "I gave birth to a seven and a half pound girl, *a la* CWF (Childbirth Without Fear). Everything came off beautifully. Total labor, two hours and 20 minutes, and it was not painful. I was up and about five and a half hours after her birth, and I feel wonderful. Doctor, I've learned a lot from your column, especially about natural childbirth, rooming-in or having one's baby at home."

One woman who has had "such a wonderful, gratifying, rewarding experience" (natural childbirth) says there is no unendurable pain and "the only thing one has to fear is fear itself."

This reminds me of the "obstetric stage" of anesthesia. We don't hear much about it nowadays. I learned about it as an intern in the County Hospital—which was so far from the offices of the staff physicians that they gave us interns a good deal more freedom to do things ourselves than interns generally are allowed. So we were the ones who delivered the babies, except when an assistant to the Professor of Obstetrics and her students, happened to visit the hospital.

Shortly after I entered practice a senior colleague called me to a patient's home, to give the anesthetic while he essayed a forceps delivery. The patient, a young woman in labor for the first time, had finished high school and one year of college. She was intelligent but uneducated. Her parents and teachers had regarded embryology, prenatal hygiene, childbirth and care of the baby as improper subjects for a teenage girl to study. Her girl friends before marriage and the fishwives after her marriage had taught her that childbirth is a dreadful ordeal. So she was terribly frightened.

The doctor explained that she had been in labor all night without making any progress so he had decided to use forceps. The patient was crying and moaning and tossing about. While the doctor busied himself sterilizing instruments, I asked if I might start the anesthetic. "Give her just a little," he said, "I'm not quite ready yet."

Just a little was all she needed—the obstetric stage of anesthesia. It took the edge off her pain, so she listened to my instructions on how to breathe between pains and bear down with the rhythmic contractions. She became quiet and settled down to her work. Before the doctor could get the forceps ready the patient finished the job herself—as she would have done hours earlier had she received a little encouragement.

I do not mean to say that childbirth is completely painless, only that many women who have experienced natural childbirth minimize the pain or even insist it does not really exist. Childbirth is a natural, physiological process, and knowledge of just what is happening robs it of its terrors.

One of the cruelties all too often inflicted on the hospital inmate is solitary isolation—the godless hospital attendants put her in a room and leave her there alone for hours, while waiting for completion of the first stage of labor—dilatation of the cervix, opening of neck or orifice of womb—at which point she can be taken to the delivery room. From time to time, as the unhappy prisoner lies there in a state of terror, some assistant nurse or probationer sticks her head in the door and asks how she's doing. Women who have been subjected to such maltreatment describe it as horrible. However the prison—I mean hospital—officials have an answer for the statement that a woman in childbirth should never be left alone. How can they take nurses away from their duties to just sit there . . . ! And of course it would be against hospital rules to let the patient's husband or a relative or friend keep her company. This cruelty is something else that does not occur in normal childbirth—childbirth at home.

The young woman who refused to listen to any discussion of natural childbirth was trying to conceal her ignorance and her fears. A good many persons who are adult in general intelligence are child-minded in respect to the whole subject of childbirth and infant care. Not merely our grade school and high school curricula, but our whole system of education is at fault here.

Ah, say some persons who haven't quite grown up, but suppose the woman required a transfusion, a Caesarian section or instrumental delivery. What could you do for her at home? The answer is that we would do whatever we considered best for her. You must remember it is no great problem nowadays to move a patient to the hospital in an emergency.

A mouthpiece for the doctors who want to make childbirth an abnormal occurrence and for hospitals that still maintain a star chamber secrecy about the delivery room, explained to a reporter who inquired about husbands remaining with their wives in the delivery room, that nurses and doctors were much too busy to take care of fainting husbands. This, I thought, was a sad commentary on American manhood.

I read somewhere just the other day that the birth of a baby hallows the home. True enough provided the baby is born at home. Yet even a little stranger born in a hospital or adopted makes a house a home.

The more you know about the baby business, if a plodding old horse-and-buggy practitioner may venture to advise young people, the less you will like the idea of going to a hospital to have your baby.

We had our own babies at home. I was on the hospital staff. Their mother was a graduate nurse. Our home was nothing fancy either—an old frame house for which we paid $20 a month rent, and later a newer frame house for which we paid $26 a month rent—we never were able to make a small down payment for a house of our own until we were about 40 years old and the children were in high school. But we had a home from that great moment, the greatest moment in our lives, when our first baby was born. We had named her about two years earlier, when her mother-to-be was the loveliest nurse I ever saw and I was an intern aged 22. We named her after her mother's mother, Elizabeth, but her younger sister never could manage that, so she called her Lalla, and Lalla called her younger sister Henny, the best she could do with Helen. They were not only born at home but their father delivered them though of course on both occasions I did have a colleague alerted to be ready to come to my assistance if I called him. I am not at all sure I could have been the accoucheur if the babies had been born in a hospital—there may have been some hospital rule or regulation prohibiting it. Hospitals are funny that way.

Once a colleague asked me to attend his wife in labor at the hospital. When she reached the second stage I called for chloroform which I had always used with the most satisfactory results. There was much scurrying about and presently a nurse came with a message from the superintendent—the hospital did not permit the use of chloroform. Only ether. I was so mad I would have taken my patient elsewhere—but I couldn't do that with a colleague's wife. Neither the patient nor her husband would have cared for a terrible-tempered Mr. Bang act in such circumstance.

Please do not get the impression that I don't like hospitals. My experience as a hospital patient, especially for surgery, has been not just pleasant but downright delightful. A well managed modern hospital is a wonderful institution for sick people—but not for people having babies.

Lately it has become the custom to send women home within 40 to 50 hours after delivery. It has been found that they get along much better if they get up shortly after childbirth and resume their activities, instead of lying abed nine days or whatever the magic number was when childbirth was and too often became an illness.

Some women chide me for urging home delivery, saying that a week or two in hospital having a baby is the only way they ever get a chance to loaf and rest from the exacting job of taking care of their young children, husband and households.

I agree that a woman with such a job deserves at least an annual two-week vacation with pay. In fact I advocate a state law providing a bonus payable to every mother upon filing the birth certificate —a sum sufficient to pay a qualified housekeeper for two weeks' service. But the mother should be able to collect only if she really does take that vacation, spending the two weeks as she likes.

There is of course one big difficulty about this plan. Many mothers just couldn't enjoy themselves—they would worry so much about the welfare of the kids and even of their father. Heck, most of them worry about the household and the family even while they are in hospital. A husband on the other hand lightly shifts any such responsibilities to his homebody wife and enjoys any vacation coming to him in manly fashion.

Still and all, I protest that women who plan to spend a week or more in hospital and doctors who send them there to have babies are abusing the hospital system. It is as wrong for a healthy young woman to occupy a hospital room or bed for a week while having a child as it is for a man to hog a room or a bed while in for "observation" or "a check-up." There is a constant cry about the shortage of nurses and hospital facilities for the sick and the injured. The pampered ones and their trick specialists should not be permitted to appropriate those facilities and services which rightly belong to those who really need them.

The sooner we stop treating childbirth as an abnormal, "delicate" or morbid condition the better it will be for potential and prospective mothers, for women in labor and for the world in general. Turn back to what women who have experienced natural childbirth say about labor pain. They minimize it. They have learned about it by reading and from instruction by qualified teachers.

It is axiomatic that we most fear the unknown.

Every boy and girl old enough to enter high school should receive at least elementary instruction in pre-natal hygiene, normal childbirth and infant care. Far better to teach them the truth at an early age while they are still under parental control than to leave their education entirely to chance.

Chapter Twenty-five

A DIAGNOSIS OF DOCTORING

In the horse and buggy era, the time of Dr. Osler, 98 out of 100 physicians were general practitioners, family physicians; two out of 100 were real specialists. A high school diploma admitted a student to medical school and many completed medical school and received the degree, Doctor of Medicine, in *three* years. This was possible up to the turn of the century. After 1900 the medical school course was standardized and ever since has been four years.

When someone with the M.D. degree passes an examination given by the State or Provincial Board of Medical Examiners and receives a license to practice in the state or province, he or she is *legally* qualified to practice medicine, surgery, obstetrics or any branch thereof. Few licensees take advantage of this defect in the law. License holders who intend to limit practice to a special field invariably take post-graduate instruction before they begin practice.

Two out of 100 physicians in horse and buggy days were specialists, I said. I mean *real* specialists—indeed that was the only kind there were then. True, probably no more than two percent of today's physicians are real specialists too, but recent surveys indicate that a new breed, the *trick* specialists, actually outnumber general practitioners or family physicians.

A real specialist limits his practice to a particular field.

A trick specialist latches onto whatever business comes his way and competes unfairly for the patronage of the public with the general practitioners in the community.

The trick specialist cashes in on the widely held and completely naive notion that a specialist must be better educated or better trained than an "ordinary" doctor. This enables him to charge the customers who flock to his sumptuous shop about three times what an honest doctor charges. But while their money lasts, the snobs love it. Only specialists are good enough for them.

Specialization became rampant only after Dr. Osler left the country to become Regius Professor of Medicine at Oxford in 1905. It seemed almost as though the merchants of medicine felt they could cut loose now that they were no longer restrained by the Osler influence.

With the rapid growth of trick specialization and in close association with it, medicine in the twentieth century also became afflicted with the "clinic" evil. In horse and buggy days a clinic was an institution where patients or out-patients were examined and treated free for the *instruction of medical students*. According to Webster, that's what *clinic* still means today. But a lot of ignorant folk think a clinic consists of a group of specialists who work on the assembly line plan, each in turn examining the customer and sending him along to the next, with all of them finally submitting their findings and views to the chief. The chief then decides what ails the customer and what is to be done about him— and hands him a memorandum to give the cashier on his way out.

The "clinic" racket and trick specialization are twin evils which tarnish the good name of medicine in the esteem of the public. Happily, reaction is beginning to set in. Phony "clinics" are now outlawed in at least one state: in 1958 the California legislature enacted a statute prohibiting the licensing of any such institution. Of course even this new law can't stop "clinics" that were in existence before it was enacted. The racket is rife in all parts of the country, perhaps because people generally think that eminent doctors can do no wrong.

Readers of my newspaper health column complain constantly how difficult it is to get a doctor to make a house call when a member of the household is taken ill. "A doctor," they say. I notice that seldom if ever does anyone complain how difficult it is to get *the family physician* on such occasions. From this I infer that they have no family physician. After all, this is the second half of the twentieth century—and who wants to piddle around with such a quaint character when for only a few dollars more you can consult a specialist or go to a "clinic?"

It takes at least ten years after high school to get a medical education today. It took less than six to get it in my day. Yet I venture to say I was as well trained as the average young doctor today. I can't see the difference between physicians who passed directly from high school into medical school and those who spend four years in college.

All this window dressing, the "clinic" setups, the so-called specialists and doctors' reluctance to visit sick people at home—to say nothing of the abuse of hospital facilities by pampered private patients with nothing to do but loll about and be waited on for a week or two while having periodic "checkups" or while "under observation"—all this, I say, only goes to show that what this country needs is 100 new medical schools to train students for *general practice as family physicians,* training them in six years from high school to M.D. degree.

We also need a legal requirement to the effect that a Doctor of Medicine shall have served a reasonable period, say five to ten years, in general practice before being permitted to call himself a specialist.

Thirty years ago I called the gullible customers $300 snobs. Today everything comes higher. So now they've become $1000 snobs. I am referring to the poor boobs who fall for the myth that a doctor who attaches the label of specialist to himself necessarily is better trained or more competent than an unpretentious GP. The $1000 snobs will, for instance, invariably pass up the lowly general practitioner in favor of an exclusive pediatrician when it comes to having babies; and once the pediatrician has a snob mother hypnotized he's booked solid to care for her offspring until the baby begins to vote. The specialist knows no more than an "ordinary" doctor about the feeding, clothing and immunization of children, but the snobs derive a lot of satisfaction from being in a position to talk about what "my pediatrician" says.

One pediatrician told me in a personal communication: "On the one hand I must say that your baby book gives excellent advice about care of the baby, but on the other hand I can't help complaining that you are queering my game . . ."

This frank avowal reminds me that the information and advice in my pocketsize baby book is merely what every youngster should be required to learn in high school. A high school course in the care and feeding of infants would make girls better wives and boys better husbands. But in Yankeeland when a young man shows interest in and capability for taking care of a baby, people still consider it humorous.

For that matter, the information and advice contained in the other pamphlets in the *Pocket Cyclopedia of Health*—the gist of the teachings in my health column—intelligently applied to problems of hygiene and illness in the home make unnecessary a good deal of expensive doctoring. A good many parents have reported, for instance, that the annual doctor bills have been substantially reduced since everyone in the family has learned how the CRI spreads. Nor do they as frequently call the doctor since learning how to whip up a batch of *Home-made Foolproof Cough Medicine* whenever a member of the family needs it.

Some druggists are plumb annoyed when a customer asks for two ounces of citrate of soda, an item in the recipe for making the cough medicine. They go so far as to refuse to sell it without a prescription or even try to tell people it is no longer obtainable or perhaps that it is too dangerous. Well, it wasn't dangerous in horse and buggy days! It was commonly used in the baby's bottle, a few grains of it to prevent curd formation. If a druggist ever does try to pull that line on you, just keep your temper and say okay, you'll settle for two ounces of potassium citrate instead. Citrate of potash serves the purpose about as well as citrate of soda. Of course if the druggist still fusses and fumes—and after all why shouldn't he since he would be making a much bigger profit on a bottle of ready-made cough medicine—you may feel free to take your patronage elsewhere.

When readers complain how difficult it is to find a doctor willing to make a house call when a member of the family is ill, I cannot help wondering whether the difficulty isn't at least in part of the public's own making. Too many people nowadays don't even know a doctor in their own neighborhood and no local doctor knows them. Unwittingly they themselves compound the evil of the specialization racket by thinking it's smart to turn to a specialist when something ails them. So of course they have no family doctor to rely on.

I am well aware that doctors do use various stratagems to avoid making house visits. Whoever answers the telephone or doorbells is very sorry, but the doctor is attending a confinement. Or if the doctor does answer himself he instructs the patient to bundle up and come to the office. If that isn't feasible he prescribes by phone, with instructions to report to him in the morning.

When a trick specialist or "clinic wizard" prescribes by telephone for a patient who is acutely ill, in my opinion he is committing malpractice. If he is unable himself to visit the patient to determine just what is wrong and what treatment is indicated, he should either send a colleague or an assistant or advise the family to call another physician. The dodge of instructing a sick child's mother to take the child's temperature, give it a dose of aspirin and report later on doesn't extenuate such malpractice. Worse still is the way some "specialists" keep the customers in line. They direct them to bundle up a child and bring it to the office, where whatever the child happens to be ill with will doubtless spread to others in the waiting room.

The merchants of medicine are great believers in advertising— not the kind you buy by the line, inch, column or page but the kind they get gratis. What made the first "clinic" famous was chiefly the willingness, I might even say the eagerness of newspapers and magazines to print thousands of pieces in praise of the institution and of the doctors who worked wonders there. There was never any allusion, of course, to the many poor souls who mortgaged their homes to pay for a trip to the "clinic"—only to find that their sacrifice had been in vain.

The great majority of Americans who patronize "clinics" are sold on them, convinced that doctors who take salaried jobs are somehow better than men who practice medicine as a private, personal service. Perhaps this conviction could be turned into a good thing.

Perhaps the public could be stirred up into demanding that we develop a lot more of what this country needs: many more *real* clinics than exist at present.

In lots of communities, towns or cities with population of around 20,000 there are excellent hospital facilities and even ambulance service available, but only or mainly for people who can pay. There is no clinic or dispensary service for those who can't. Yet a hospital without a bona fide clinic and dispensary for people who cannot afford private care cannot be considered a *public* hospital.

And now I have a confession to make. Over the past 25 years we have learned to put great faith in our own family doctor. (Oh, yes, I learned long ago that a doctor had better not try to treat members of his own family; I even lean far over backward to give the outsider we call in absolute authority when he is treating a member of my household). When this man gives us his opinion or advice we are content to accept it as probably correct and we've never sought any other doctor's judgment except with his approval. I take credit for having discovered this particular doctor, although for the life of me I can no longer remember how I happened to consult him in the first place. I remember only that I was greatly impressed by the methodical, scientific way he went about examining me—just the way I like to imagine Dr. Osler would have done it.

Well, sir, four or five years after he first started treating us I was painfully shocked by the announcement that he had quit private practice and with a number of his colleagues organized and set up in business as the _____ Clinic. If not its actual head, he was certainly the leader around whom the venture grew. His name on the roster gives the outfit an air of respectability. I felt sad about our doctor's dereliction but didn't lose faith in him. He is still our first thought whenever we need medical advice or treatment.

I am well aware of the pressure *our* doctor was under. There are others in the same predicament. This I know from what they tell me. The other day, for instance, I received a note on the letterhead of a fancy "clinic" in the midwest, signed by its medical director, congratulating me on my educating the public in reference to this whole racket! He fervently wished he were out of it, he said. But he hasn't the courage to get out. He then put a question to me that has given me furiously to think: Could I consider giving up my newspaper column and go back to my little old practice in Penn Yan or Elmira?

Now this is odd. Up to now I have often dreamed of doing just that—of hanging up my shingle at the old stand and trying to make a living as an honest family doctor. The dream has always been a pleasant one. But now I'm afraid my "clinic"-bound colleague has spoiled it for me. The very thought of relinquishing the soft berth where I have lolled happily for the past 47 years and going back to real work—even with a bowling green included in the deal —sounds dreadful and unthinkable. Of course, it is entirely possible I may be out of the health column racket altogether in another year or two whether I like it or not; but that would be courtesy of the cheat-food vendors, and the big nostrum makers, all of whom sound rather anxious to silence me. It seems my teachings annoy them. So I may have no choice in the matter.

Before the merchants of medicine converted the profession into a business, it was a comfort to know the physician you called to attend a member of your family in an emergency was a friend who knew the patient's history and would be ready to help—ready *and* willing. Nowadays your frantic midnight call reaches a switchboard operator who tells you in a mechanical tone that she will try to reach the doctor who will then get in touch with you. Except on Wednesdays and weekends, of course, which he reserves for recreation. . . .

Well, in all fairness you can't expect the doctor to be on duty and on call 24 hours a day, seven days a week. He is human too and needs time off even more than, say, a bus driver. But just as the bus passengers have a right to feel confident that when their driver goes home for the night or the weekend they will not be left stranded on a street corner, so the doctor has a special obligation to arrange for someone to take his place and be available when he himself isn't around. In some communities doctors do arrange for weekend, holiday, emergency or night service by taking turns on call. In too many other places, however, no such happy arrangement is possible because the doctors are too distrustful of one another.

There is another reason for the existing situation: Reliable round-the-clock medical service is not profitable—it is not the kind of business the merchants of medicine welcome. The reluctance to answer hurry calls at odd hours has become widespread since medicine has been converted from a profession to a business.

Yet I know of at least one group of doctors calling themselves a "clinic" who mail out telephone stickers saying the clinic has doctors on duty 24 hours a day for emergency service. Remember, this is not a public or charity service but strictly business. Well, if a phony "clinic" can advertise in this manner, why shouldn't the doctors in any community set up a similar plan for taking care of hurry calls.

ONE LAST WORD: If you are fortunate enough to have a doctor who is devoted to healing and reassurance, hang onto him and treat him gently, for you can hardly find his kind any more. The horse and buggy may be gone with the wind, but not the need for the family doctor.

INDEX